Cleofina Bosco
Eugenia Diaz

ALCOHOL EXPOSURE EFFECTS IN PLACENTAL HYPOXIA AND FETAL DEVELOPMENT

Cleofina Bosco
Eugenia Diaz

ALCOHOL EXPOSURE EFFECTS IN PLACENTAL HYPOXIA AND FETAL DEVELOPMENT

Alcoholism in pregnancy

LAP LAMBERT Academic Publishing

Impressum / Imprint

Bibliografische Information der Deutschen Nationalbibliothek: Die Deutsche Nationalbibliothek verzeichnet diese Publikation in der Deutschen Nationalbibliografie; detaillierte bibliografische Daten sind im Internet über http://dnb.d-nb.de abrufbar.
Alle in diesem Buch genannten Marken und Produktnamen unterliegen warenzeichen-, marken- oder patentrechtlichem Schutz bzw. sind Warenzeichen oder eingetragene Warenzeichen der jeweiligen Inhaber. Die Wiedergabe von Marken, Produktnamen, Gebrauchsnamen, Handelsnamen, Warenbezeichnungen u.s.w. in diesem Werk berechtigt auch ohne besondere Kennzeichnung nicht zu der Annahme, dass solche Namen im Sinne der Warenzeichen- und Markenschutzgesetzgebung als frei zu betrachten wären und daher von jedermann benutzt werden dürften.

Bibliographic information published by the Deutsche Nationalbibliothek: The Deutsche Nationalbibliothek lists this publication in the Deutsche Nationalbibliografie; detailed bibliographic data are available in the Internet at http://dnb.d-nb.de.
Any brand names and product names mentioned in this book are subject to trademark, brand or patent protection and are trademarks or registered trademarks of their respective holders. The use of brand names, product names, common names, trade names, product descriptions etc. even without a particular marking in this works is in no way to be construed to mean that such names may be regarded as unrestricted in respect of trademark and brand protection legislation and could thus be used by anyone.

Coverbild / Cover image: www.ingimage.com

Verlag / Publisher:
LAP LAMBERT Academic Publishing
ist ein Imprint der / is a trademark of
OmniScriptum GmbH & Co. KG
Heinrich-Böcking-Str. 6-8, 66121 Saarbrücken, Deutschland / Germany
Email: info@lap-publishing.com

Herstellung: siehe letzte Seite /
Printed at: see last page
ISBN: 978-3-659-57399-6

Copyright © 2014 OmniScriptum GmbH & Co. KG
Alle Rechte vorbehalten. / All rights reserved. Saarbrücken 2014

TABLE OF CONTENT

Highlights	3
Introduction	5
Processes in the embryonic development	6
Functions of the placenta	7
Placenta and oxidative stress	11
Peroxynitrite mediates placental lipid oxidation and nitration	14
Apoptosis in the placenta	19
Fetal development and oxidative stress	22
Alcohol and hypertension in pregnancy	26
Impaired placentation in rat fetal alcohol syndrome	27
Hypoxic stress and neuroactive steroid responses	28
Alcohol-induced neural crest cells apoptosis	31
Alterations in brain and behaviour by fetal alcohol exposure	33
Effect of alcohol on cardiac embryo development	37
Effect of alcohol on liver embryo development	38
Effect of alcohol on lung embryo development	39
Summary and conclusions	41
References	43

HIGHLIGHTS

Sustained alcohol abuse by pregnant women is clearly on the rise, so their effects on pregnancy outcomes are today considered important public health issues. Alcohol is one of the commonest teratogenic agents and its uncontrolled consumption by pregnant women can give rise to an irreversible condition in the child called Fetal Alcohol Spectrum Disorders (FASD). Cases that exhibit all of the following criteria: central nervous system dysfunction, prenatal and postnatal growth deficiency and cranial/facial abnormalities, are referred as fetal alcohol syndrome (FAS). All children of mothers who abuse alcohol consumption during pregnancy do not necessarily develop FAS/FASD. The potential source of individual variability includes differences in the pattern, frequency and duration of the period of drinking, differences in maternal, fetal and placental metabolism of ethanol/acetaldehyde, as well as genetic factors. Studies performed in animal models suggest that acetaldehyde, the primary hepatic oxidative metabolite of ethanol, reaches the foetus either by placental production or by placental transference, which in turn could affect fetal growth and development. The most likely hypothesis regarding the decrease of fetal growth is thought to be via hypoxia and increased oxidative stress, both of which interfere with cellular processes that require oxygen in order to function adequately, such as placental transport. This review summarizes recent findings on placental hypoxia, oxidative/nitrative stress and fetal development that may play a role in the impairment of essential fetal metabolites that could be related to FAS/FASD syndrome.

INTRODUCTION

The fetotoxic effects of maternal alcohol consumption have been widely documented for over three decades, but the mechanisms underlying this devastating phenomenon remain uncertain. In most women, the recognition of the pregnancy condition does not occur until 4 to 6 weeks of gestation (Floyd et al., 1999), and thus many women may drink alcohol prior to realizing they are pregnant. Upon recognition of pregnancy most women spontaneously reduce their alcohol intake. Hence, fetal alcohol exposure prior to and after pregnancy outcomes are important public health concerns (Floyd et al., 2009). The wide variety of cellular/biochemical effects of alcohol on fetal tissues strongly suggests that the fetotoxic responses to alcohol may reflect a multifactorial setting. Many of these responses can be conceptually connected to effects on the structure and function of the cellular plasmatic membrane (Henderson et al., 1999).

Alcohol is one of the commonest teratogenic agents and its uncontrolled consumption by pregnant women can give rise to an irreversible condition in the child called Fetal Alcohol Syndrome (FAS) (Fukui and Fakata-Haga (2009). This syndrome, described earlier by Jones and Smith (1973), is characterized by intrauterine growth retardation (IUGR), craniofacial malformations, physical and mental retardation, motor incoordination, and cardiac septal defects (American Academy of Pediatrics, 2000). However, FAS represents only a part of the spectrum of fetal alcohol effects. In this regard, fetal alcohol spectrum disorders (FASD) is a term currently used to describe a lesser degree of deformities associated to FAS, sometimes unnoticeable except by close examination and usually related to a variable degree of mental retardation (Rosett, 1980; Chaudhuri, 2000). While some offspring of mothers who drink heavily during pregnancy develop FAS and shown all the symptoms described above, some others show no symptoms at all, a condition known as ethanol resilience (Gemma et al., 2006; Gemma et al., 2007), while many more show only partial FAS-related phenotypes. It has been proposed that maternal ethanol ingestion may cause fetal injury and impairment of somatic and brain growth, by at least two mechanisms: i) directly, by fetotoxicity from ethanol and/or acetaldehyde; ii) indirectly, by ethanol induced placental injury and selective foetal malnutrition (Fisher and Karl, 1988; Bosco, 2005).

All together, these findings suggest that environmental and genetic factors from the foetal compartment may confer a certain degree of vulnerability or resilience to ethanol-induced teratogenesis. It has been observed that certain tissues, organs or systems appear to be more vulnerable than others are, depending on dose, duration and timing of exposure to alcohol (Gemma et al., 2007; Giles et al., 2008; Salihu et al, 2011, Shaukat et al., 2011). Accurate information regarding the risks of alcohol consumption during pregnancy is needed in order to support the efforts aimed to the design and implementation of programs of health promotion and prevention strategies (Gahagan et al., 2006). In order to contribute to a better understanding of the teratogenic effects of alcohol, this review will focus on recent insights into the normal process of placental and human development susceptible to be affected by alcohol consumption during pregnancy.

PROCESSES IN THE EMBRYONIC DEVELOPMENT

The human embryo originates from the fertilization of the oocyte by the sperm at the oviduct. After fertilization, the nuclei of the sperm and the oocyte fuse to form a new cell (the zygote). This cell contains 46 chromosomes, 23 from each parental cell. As the zygote travels to the uterus, it divides, forming a cluster of cells (morula) by about 3 days after fertilization. As the morula enters the uterine cavity, fluid penetrates into it to form the blastocyst. The epithelial outer wall of this structure constitute the trophoblast, and the inner cell mass the embryoblast. During implantation, the trophoblast differentiates into two layers, the syncytiotrophoblast and the cytotrophoblast. Mitchell and Goldman (1996) demonstrates in the rat that alcohol, at a dose comparable to social drinking in man, alters uterine vascular perfusion. Uterine blood flow is markedly increased and the perfusion of the vascular bed developing at sites of blastocyst implantation is significantly enhanced. Such haemodynamic effects of alcohol are consistent with its ability to influence blastocyst implantation, embrionic development and endometrial decidualization in the rat.

In the blastocyst, the syncytiotrophoblast constitutes the external layer and has multiple nuclei and a continuous cytoplasm forming a syncytium. The cytotrophoblast consists of a layer of ovoid cells, located immediately under the syncytiotrophoblast. Both structures contribute to the formation of the villi and ultimately the placenta. During placentation, cytotrophoblast cells localized in floating and anchoring villi follow distinct differentiation pathways (Cross et al., 1994 : a) Villous cytotrophoblast fuse to form the syncytiotrophoblast layer that contributes to the exchange of gas and nutrient, as well as waste elimination, so villous syncytiotrophoblast provides the epithelial cover of the placental villous trees in direct contact to maternal blood (Bosco and Díaz, 2012). In recent years, the fusion between cytotrophoblast and the overlying multinucleate syncytiotrophoblast is considered as the apoptotic event of the syncytiotrophoblast (Heasell and Crocker (2008). b) In anchoring villi, cytotrophoblast generates a multilayered column of highly invasive extravillous trophoblast (EVT). This EVT invades maternal uterine tissues thus directly contacting maternal stromal and immune cells (Huppertz et al, 2006) and later migrate into the decidua and remodels the endometrial spiral arteries to produce the low-resistance vascular system that is essential for fetal growth (Pijnenborg et al., 1981a, 1981b; Aplin, 1991; Huppertz et al, 2006). One characteristic feature of serious conditions such as preeclampsia or IUGR is the occurrence of changes in apoptosis regulation in villous and/or EVT resulting in altered trophoblast invasion and/or shedding into the maternal circulation.

Human embryogenesis takes place in a hypoxic environment because the trophoblast shell excludes the entry of considerable amount of maternal blood. Due to the fact that the early conceptus has little protection against oxygen-generated free radicals, this low-oxygen environment is essential for normal embryonic and placental development. The first fetal-placental villi develop as trophoblast sprouts, which are subsequently invaded by extraembryonic mesoderm to form secondary villi and are transformed, by vasculogenesis, into tertiary villi. The placental barrier to maternal blood becomes gradually breached at about 8-12 weeks of gestation, due to the invasion of placental-bed uteroplacental spiral arteries by the EVT, and consequently placental oxygen tension significantly rise (Kingdom and Kaufmann, 1999). This developmental period is characterized by an important physiological switch of the oxygen tension at the opening of the intervillous space (Genbacev et al., 1997).

As development proceeds, the embryoblast cell mass organizes itself into a flat disc-shaped structure, the bilaminar germ disc, which consists of two layers of cells, the epiblast and the hypoblast, with the primitive streak forming ulterior on the surface of the epiblast. During the gastrulation process, the cells of the epiblast layer migrate towards the primitive streak to form the mesoderm layer between the epiblast layer and the hypoblast layer forming the trilaminar germ disc, composed by ectoderm, mesoderm and endoderm germ layers. These three layers are responsible for the formation of all the body organ systems. The ectodermal germ layer gives rise to the nervous system, the retina of the eye and the epidermal layer of the skin. The mesoderm germ layer gives rise to the cardiovascular system and most part of the musculoskeletal system and the genitourinary system. The endoderm germ layer gives rise to the gastrointestinal system.

Alcohol effects on the described developmental processes probably occur through multiple mechanisms and a range of disabilities has been observed in the absence of dysmorphic features, reflecting variable degrees of damage during fetal development. It is reasonable to assume that both the timing and the degree of alcohol exposure are important factors that contribute to this variation (Chudley et al., 2005). An important but yet unresolved question is when exactly the critical periods for ethanol exposure are manifested during embryogenesis, and which of the molecular components that are expressed during such periods are ethanol-sensitive.

This issue is difficult to establish with precision in mammalian embryos inside the womb, even more given the variations existing within and among litters (Kaufman, 1992).

FUNCTIONS OF THE PLACENTA

The passage of nutrients from the maternal blood to the foetus is mediated by the placenta, an organ that establishes critical functional connections for embryonic survival (Cross et al., 1994). The placenta mediates the process of implantation and establishes the interface for both nutrient and gas exchange between the maternal and fetal circulation. It also plays a key role on maternal recognition of pregnancy, altering the immune environment and the maternal cardiovascular and metabolic functions through the production of paracrine and endocrine hormones (Cross, 2006). The placenta transports oxygen, nutrients and antibodies to the foetus by means of the umbilical vein; removes carbon dioxide and metabolic waste from the foetus by the two umbilical arteries; serves as a protective barrier against harmful effects produced by certain drugs and microorganisms; acts as a partial barrier between the mother and foetus in order to prevent fetal and maternal blood from mixing; and produces steroid and peptide hormones essential for maintaining the pregnancy: estrogen, progesterone, and human chorionic gonadotropin (hCG) (Bosco, 1995; Bosco 2005). Normal fetal metabolism and growth require an adequate exchange across the placenta. The barrier that separates maternal and fetal blood in the human placenta is classified as villous hemomonochorial and it is composed of one layer of trophoblast and the fetal capillary endothelium (Enders, 1965; Bosco, 1994).

Epigenetic regulation of the placenta evolves during the preimplantation developmental period and further gestation. Epigenetic modification refers to heritable changes in gene expression that are not mediated by alterations in DNA sequence (Jaenisch and Bird, 2003). Epigenetic markers, like DNA methylation, histone modifications and non-coding RNAs, affect gene expression patterns. These expression patterns, including the important parent-of-origin-dependent gene expression resulting from genomic imprinting, play a pivotal role in proper fetal and placental development. Imprinted genes are those whose expression depends on their parental origin. In a paternally imprinted gene, for example, the maternal allele is silenced by DNA methylation (Delaval and Feil, 2004). Imprinting is also controlled by epigenetic mechanisms under the control of environmental factors and nutrients (Reik et al., 2003). This may provide a linkage between maternal nutrition and fetal placental growth (Myatt, 2006).

Disturbed placental epigenetics has been demonstrated in cases of IUGR and small for gestational age (SGA), and appears to be involved in the pathogenesis of pre-eclampsia (PE) and gestational trophoblastic disease. Several environmental effects have been investigated so far, e.g. ethanol, oxygen tension as well as the effect of several aspects of assisted reproduction technologies on placental epigenetics. Studies carried out in both animal models and humans have made it increasingly clear that proper epigenetic regulation of both imprinted and non-imprinted genes is important in placental development. Its disturbance, which can be caused by various environmental factors, can lead to abnormal placental development and function with possible consequences for maternal morbidity, fetal development and disease susceptibility in later life, (Nelissen et al., 2011).

It is widely known that the number of placental genes altered by moderate ethanol exposure plays critical roles in pattern formation during nervous system development. For example, interactions of some members of the transforming growth factor b (TGFb) family, such as the bone morphogenic protein 4 (BMP4) and the BMP4 antagonist chordin, help to regulate polarity in the establishment of dorso-ventral patterning of the developing embryo (Chesnutt et al., 2004; Millet et al., 2001). Considerable work remains to be done in order to confirm the utility of placental gene alterations as a biomarker system, both for detecting ethanol consumption and a prognostic indicator of adverse neurobehavioral outcomes in the absence of morphological alterations. Systematic examination of altered gene expression as a function of different levels and patterns of ethanol consumption, as well as the persistence of gene alterations after the last drinking episode are critical questions that remain to be addressed. Further, how the presence of other common pregnancy risk factors influences ethanol-induced alterations in placental gene expression patterns needs to be determined. For example, how will concomitant exposure to such factors as nicotine, other drugs of abuse, stress, malnutrition, or heavy metals exposure, modify a biomarker signature pattern? Data from such studies would be critical for interpreting altered patterns of placental gene expression in clinical studies (Rosenberg et al., 2010). An earlier review addressing the fetal consequences of ethanol-induced disruption of placental transport of nutrients, hypoxia, and calcium-handling mechanisms pinpointed the distribution of ethanol onto the lipid membrane of the placental cell as one agent affecting the action of ion channels and proteins (Michaelis, 1990). Furthermore, the placenta generates reactive oxygen species (ROS) which may contribute to the oxidative stress observed even in normal pregnancy, but this is increased in pregnancies complicated by PE, IUGR and pregestational diabetes, where oxidative stress and nitrative stress are increased (Webster et al., 2008; Myatt, 2010).

In humans, the occurrence of prenatal exposure to ethanol is difficult to validate objectively. In order to assess intrauterine exposure to alcohol, increased concentration of fatty acid ethyl ester (FAEE) and the presence of non-oxidative ethanol metabolites in the meconium of the newborn has been proposed as a novel screening method (Chan et al., 2004, Brien et al., 2006). Recently, it has been demonstrated that identical maternal ethanol exposure levels produced different levels of fetal exposure in a dizygotic human twin pair. This was also observed in guinea pig littermates through FAEE meconium analysis. The authors concluded that the placenta may have a previously unappreciated role in mediating ethanol-induced fetal injury (Gareri et al., 2009).

PLACENTA AND OXIDATIVE STRESS

Placental pathology has long been associated with IUGR and PE in humans. The development of the placenta is a highly regulated process and is therefore quite susceptible to perturbation. Several genetic, epigenetic, nutritional and environmental factors associated with complications in pregnancy outcome, ranging from embryonic lethality to fetal growth restriction, have been identified (Myllynen et al., 2005; Cross, 2006). A variety of factors may interfere with placental functions at many levels including cell signalling, production and release of hormones and enzymes, transport of nutrients and waste products, implantation, cellular growth and maturation, and finally in the delivery. Placental responses may also be due to alcohol/toxicodynamic responses, e.g. hypoxia (Myllynen et al., 2005). On the other hand, oxidative stress constitutes a unifying mechanism of injury of many types of disease processes. It occurs when there is an imbalance between the production of ROS and the ability of the biological system to readily detoxify these reactive intermediates or easily repair the resulting damage (Rodrigo et al., 2005). ROS such as hydrogen peroxide and hydroxyl radicals are formed via a variety of physiological and pathophysiological reactions, and its formation can be enhanced by xenobiotics (Wells et al., 2009). The mechanism of oxidative stress seems to operate in alcohol ingest pregnancy (Ornoy, 2007) and it has also been demonstrated that ethanol exposure induces oxidative stress in the human placental villi, which may account for the decreased nitric oxide (NO) release, because NO may be shunted toward scavenging free radicals (Kay et al., 2000; Dotsch et al., 2001). These authors concluded that increased endothelial nitric oxide synthase (eNOS) protein expression may be a response to the increased demand for NO. Decreased NO availability could adversely affect placental blood flow regulation which could, in turn, account for the restriction of growth observed in ethanol-exposed fetuses.

Pregnancy in itself is a condition of increased susceptibility to oxidative stress, leading to potential tissue damage (Sies, 1991). Several organs in pregnant women show increased basal oxygen consumption and changes in substrate energy use. The production of ROS within the fetal–placental unit has special relevance due to its highly vascularised nature and because the tissue is rich in mitochondria, there is an abundance of macrophages. At pregnancy term, the human placenta is hemomonochorial, i.e, only one chorionic trophoblast cell layer exists between maternal and fetal blood (Bosco 1994), thus favouring the exchange of gases, nutrients, and metabolic products. In turn, oxygen delivery is favoured by the lower partial pressure of oxygen, which raises lactic acid production and lowers pH, within the placental cells and fetal circulation. In addition, as the hypoxic placenta matures, vascularization develops to create an oxygen-rich environment (Bosco, 2005). Moreover, the increasing mitochondrial mass favours the production of ROS (Liochev and Fridovich, 1997). NO is also produced by the placenta (Dotsch et al., 2001; Bosco et al., 2012), giving rise to another local source of free radicals, likely contributing to endothelial dysfunction. In addition, the placenta is also rich in macrophages (Hofbauer cells), the local source of free radicals, including reactive chlorine species. All these chemical species might also contribute to the development of oxidative stress (Myatt and Cui, 2004). This view is based on the ability of Hofbauer cells to express both inducible nitric oxide synthase (iNOS) activity (Myatt et al., 1997) and NADPH oxidase activity (Matsubara et al., 2001), although studies on xanthine oxidase are still lacking. On the other hand, the defence mechanisms against ROS damage are also enhanced in pregnancy. Thus, a progressive increase in free radical scavengers, such as glutathione and bilirubin, as well as in the activity of antioxidant enzymes in placenta has been reported (Watson et al., 1997; Qanungo and Mukherjea, 2000).

Gundogan et al., (2010) demonstrated the impact of ethanol-mediated oxidative stress on placental trophoblast function and the potential impact on pregnancy loss. They found that rat chronically exposed to ethanol during gestation evidenced placental apoptosis/necrosis mediated through p21, Bax, and Bak via a p53-independent pathway. Ethanol mediates its adverse effect on pregnancy maintenance via inhibition of the prolactin (PRL) family hormones (placental lactogen 1 and placental lactogen 2). Prolactin receptor (PRLR) is expressed by the uterine decidual cells (Gu et al., 1996) and interacts with PRL hormones to transmit signals that mediated trophoblastic cell functions needed to maintain pregnancy (Soares, 2004). Ethanol can be placentotoxic, impairing the normal transfer of amino acids, zinc, and glucose, (Fisher and Karl, 1988). Such restriction could occur regardless of maternal nutritional status, which is known as selective fetal malnutrition (Fisher et al., 1982). Finally, it is important to consider that perturbations in the maternal compartment may affect the methylation status of placental genes and thus increase placental oxidative/nitrative stress resulting in changes in placental function (Jansson and Powell, 2007).

PEROXYNITRITE MEDIATES PLACENTAL LIPID OXIDATION AND NITRATION

As the human fetal-placental vasculature lacks autonomic innervation, autocrine and or paracrine agents such as NO radical play an important role in the regulation of fetal-placental blood flows (Myatt and Cui, 2004). This agent has been shown to maintain low-basal tone and attenuate the vasocontrictive effects of both thromboxane and endothelin (Myatt et al., 1992, Kossenjan et al., 2000). However, NO is inactivated by the superoxide anion (O_2^-), therefore limiting its activity. Conversely, the activity of NO is prolonged by the presence of superoxide dismutase (SOD) which removes superoxide. The latter is produced in living cells by NADPH oxidase, xantine oxidase, flavin enzymes and other enzymes in the mitochondrial electron transport chain. The reactivity due to the unpaired electron in superoxide leads to the production of other ROS, including the hydroxyl radical and hydrogen peroxide (Myatt et al., 1996; Myatt and Cui, 2004).

The action of superoxide *per se* is limited by its low lipid solubility, limited membrane transport and by its removal by SOD. Nevertheless, when tissues are induced to simultaneously produce both NO and superoxide in a concentrated and localized manner by inflammatory stimuli, sepsis and ischemia/reperfusion, NO and superoxide react to produce the peroxynitrite anion ($ONOO^-$). This chemical agent is a powerful oxidant of a variety of biomolecules (Beckman et al., 1994) with cytotoxic activity and inhibits mitochondrial electron transport, resulting in inhibition of cellular respiration (Radi et al., 1994). Under physiological conditions, the production of peroxynitrite will be low and oxidative damage will be minimized by endogenous antioxidant defences (Radi et al, 2002). ONOO- is extremely unstable and consequently undetectable; the evidence of its formation *in vivo* has been indirect, via the occurrence of nitrated moieties including nitrated lipids, nitrated nucleotides and nitrotyrosine residues in proteins (Pacher et al., 2007; Bosco et al., 2012). It reacts with a variety of biomolecules including proteins, lipids and DNA and can cause DNA damage by introducing oxidative modifications in the nucleobases as well as in the sugar-phosphate backbone (Burney, 1999). It is also a potent trigger of DNA strand breakage, with subsequent activation of the nuclear enzyme poly-ADP ribosyl synthetase (PARP), which causes a considerable energy depletion and necrosis of the cells (Szabó, 2003). In addition, peroxynitrite cause lipid peroxidation (Radi et al., 1991), direct inhibition of the mitochondrial electron transporter system and nitrate tyrosine residues (Brown and Borutaite, 1999; Palacios-Callender, 2004), inactivation of membrane sodium channels and oxydize sulfhydril groups on proteins, hence altering their activity or disrupting signal transduction pathways (Ischropoulos et al., 1992) and the induction of cell death through both apoptotic and necrotic mechanisms (Virag et al, 2003). It has also been demonstrated that peroxynitrite interacts with proteins via direct oxidative reactions or via indirect mechanisms radical-mediated (Pacher et al., 2007). Peroxynitrite may reach mitochondria from extramitochondrial compartments or may be directly produced within the organelle. A major physiological function of NO in the mitochondria is to regulate oxygen consumption by reversibly inhibiting cytochrome-*c* oxidase (complex IV of the electron transport chain) via competition with oxygen for the binuclear binding site (Palacios-Callender, 2004). In conditions of high NO production (e.g., during inflammation, reperfusion injury or neuronal hyperactivation), the interruption of electron transfer at cytochrome oxidase markedly increases the leakage of electrons from the respiratory chain, resulting in enhanced formation of superoxide within the mitochondrial matrix and generation of significant amounts of peroxynitrite (Brown and Borutaite, 1999). The study of MacMillan-Crow and Thompson, (1999) demonstrated that peroxynitrite is the only known biological oxidant competent to inactivate enzymatic activity, nitrate critical tyrosine residues, and induce dityrosine formation in manganese-SOD.

The production of oxidants is a crucial mechanism through which neutrophils and macrophages cause damage or kill microorganisms. When peroxynitrite acts as an oxidant, it produces nitrite and hydroxide ion rather than isomerizing to nitrate. Consequently, the major decomposition products of superoxide and peroxynitrite formation in the phagosome are ultimately hydrogen peroxide and nitrite. Within a neutrophil or macrophage phagolysosome, these reactions serve as a recycling mechanism to reutilize nitrite and hydrogen peroxide to generate more chemically reactive species. The latter are also substrates for myeloperoxidase and can be a significant source of tyrosine nitration (Burner et al., 2000) because myeloperoxidase reacts rapidly and directly with peroxynitrite to produce nitrogen dioxide and efficiently catalyzes tyrosine nitration (Floris et al., 1993). In recent years, it has become common to use nitrotyrosine as a cellular marker of nitrosative stress. Nitrotyrosine has been shown to be localized in human atherosclerotic lesions, vascular muscle (Beckmann et al., 1994) and recently in endothelial cells (Dickhout et al., 2005). In addition, Myatt et al., (1996, 2010) observed increased expression of nitrotirosine residues in the fetal vasculature and villous stroma of preeclamptic and diabetic placentas.

Disabling of several cytoskeletal proteins by nitration represents a further major cytotoxic effect attributed to peroxynitrite (Pacher et al., 2007). Tubulin nitration by peroxynitrite or by direct incorporation of free nitrotyrosine has been reported in cell lines derived from intestine (Banan et al., 2000), neurons (Tedeschi, 2005) and muscle (Chang, 2002), resulting in all the cases in loss of normal physiological functions. Peroxynitrite has also been shown to disorganizes actin polymerization through actin nitration, and via the nitration of profiling (Kasina et al, 2005), an important actin-binding protein. These effects have been associated to platelet dysfunction (Kasina et al, 2006), disruption of both intestinal (Banan et al, 2001) and endothelial barrier function (Neumann et al, 2006), as well as impaired migration and phagocytosis of activated polymorphonuclear cells (Clements et al., 2003). It is important to note that the placenta plays a function similar to that of the intestine in order to absorb metabolites and it has also been demonstrated that peroxynitrite produce intestinal barrier dysfunction mediate by ethanol-induced microtubule disruption (Banan et al., 2000). Bosco et al. (2012) have reported abundance of nitrotyrosine residues in human PE placental tissue.

The placenta is an organ with a large surface dedicated to the exchange of metabolites, and a major aspect of peroxynitrite-dependent cytotoxicity is related to its ability to trigger lipid peroxidation in membranes (Radi et al., 1991), liposomes, and lipoproteins, by the remotion of a hydrogen atom from polyunsaturated fatty acids (PUFA). Resulting products of this process include lipid hydroperoxyradicals, conjugated dienes, and aldehydes (Denicola, 2005). Such radicals in turn attack neighboring PUFAs, generating additional radicals which propagate free radical reactions and the degeneration of membrane lipids (Radi et al., 1991), causing membrane permeability and fluidity changes with significant biological consequences. Peroxynitrite may play a critical role in inflammatory diseases of the nervous system by initiating peroxidation of myelin lipids, leading to ulterior demyelination (Shi, 1999).

Once the level of cellular damage inflicted by peroxynitrite supersedes any possibility of repair, the cell eventually dies via one of the two main pathways of cell demise, necrosis or apoptosis. Necrosis is associated with loss of cellular ATP, leading to membrane disruption, release of noxious cellular debris and the development of secondary tissue inflammation. In contrast, apoptosis occurs in a well-choreographed sequence of morphological events characterized by nuclear and cytoplasmic condensation with blebbing of the plasma membrane. The dying cell eventually breaks up into apoptotic bodies, i.e., membrane-enclosed particles that are rapidly ingested and degraded by phagocytes or neighboring cells, without inducing any inflammatory response. Apoptosis is orchestrated by the proteolytic activation of cysteine proteases known as caspases that require preserved ATP levels to proceed properly, and which may be triggered either by the activation of death receptors (extrinsic pathway) or by the permeabilization of the outer membrane of mitochondria (intrinsic pathway) (Newmeyer and Ferguson-Miller, 2003). Several mechanisms have been proposed to explain the activation of the apoptotic program by peroxynitrite, which appear largely dependent on the cell type and the experimental conditions (Virag et al., 2003). However, a common pathway involving the permeabilization of the outer mitochondrial membrane is emerging as a key feature of peroxynitrite-mediated apoptosis. Whereas apoptosis is a typical consequence of low to moderate concentrations of peroxynitrite, the exposure of cells to higher concentrations of this oxidant agent has been associated with necrosis (Bonfoco et al., 1995; Virag et al., 2003).

Studies investigating the processes mentioned above have established that peroxynitrite-dependent cell necrosis is not a purely passive phenomenon, but instead is mediated by a complex process involving DNA damage and activation of the DNA repair enzyme poly [ADP-ribose] polymerase 1 (PARP-1) (Szabo et al., 1996). It has also been demonstrated that peroxynitrite selectively inactivates the prostacyclin receptor in endothelial cells (Zou et al., 1999) and decreases the amount of prostacyclin synthase through a mechanism mediated by the nuclear factor kappa-B (NF-κB) (Cooke and Davidge, 2002). NF-κB is a transcription factor involved in the enhancement of the expression of various proinflammatory biochemical markers including cytokines, chemokines and cellular adhesion molecules (Baeuerle and Henkel, 1994; Baldwin, 1996). An inactive form of NF-κB is normally present in the cytoplasm, bound to inhibitory proteins, the IκBs. The first step in this cascade is the activation of cytoplasmic inactive dimmers of NF-κB, which are bound to IκB. The critical step in NFκB activation relies on its dissociation from the IκB protein, secondary to phosphorylation and proteasomal degradation of IκB. The IκBs proteins are phosphorylated by a protein kinase complex, IκB kinase (IKK). The classical pathway of NFκB activation depends mainly on IKKβ and triggers transcription of inflammatory and antiapoptotic genes (Chen et al., 2003, Bonizzi et al., 2004). The unbound dimmers so formed are translocated into the nucleus, bind to DNA, and activate inflammatory genes. The alternative pathway, which is dependent on IKKα, has been shown to be important for B-cell maturation and lymphoid organ development (Senftleben et al., 2001). Olney et al, (2002) reported that a single episode of ethanol intoxication, lasting for several hours, triggers a massive wave of apoptotic neurodegeneration in the developing rat or mouse brain. The window of vulnerability coincides with the developmental period of synaptogenesis, also known as the brain growth-spurt period, which in rodents is a postnatal event, but in humans extends from the six month of gestation to several years after birth, (Ikonomidou et al., 2000).

APOPTOSIS IN THE PLACENTA

The morphological architecture and function of the human placenta depends on an adequate balance of proliferation, differentiation and apoptosis. In placentas from early pregnancy cell proliferation, especially of cytotrophoblasts, is very high, and decreases constantly along the duration of pregnancy (Ishihara et al., 2000). In contrast, the rate of apoptosis is low throughout early pregnancy and only increases shortly before delivery (Smith et al., 1997). The maintenance of the homeostasis of these basic processes in the placenta is a necessary condition for adequate growth and development of the foetus (Bosco and Díaz, 2012). An imbalance may result in spontaneous abortion, PE, preterm delivery and reduced fetal growth (Myatt, 2002; Crocker et al., 2003). In the last decade Huppertz et al (2006) have characterised the role of the apoptosis cascade in villous trophoblast turnover and syncytium formation. Their observations indicate that the process of syncytial fusion is linked to the "initiator stages" of the apoptosis cascade within the cytotrophoblast cells, whereas the extrusion of syncytial knots from the syncytiotrophoblast is the result of the final "execution stages" of the apoptosis cascade within the syncytiotrophoblast (Huppertz et al., 1998; Black et al., 2004). The balance between pro- and anti-apoptotic proteins determines whether apoptosis will be triggered or not.

The family of caspase proteins includes intracellular proteases termed cysteine aspartases or caspases, which cleave their targets next to an aspartic acid residue. On the basis of structural homologies and substrate preferences, the family of caspases has been subdivided into subfamilies. All the members of the subfamily of the caspase 3-like caspases (caspases 3, 6, 7, 8, 9, and 10) play central roles in the apoptosis cascade (Huppertz et al., 2006; Miller, 1997). This subfamily is further divided into signalling/initiator caspases 8, 9, and 10 and effector/execution caspases 3, 6, and 7, 12 and 13. The major difference between members of these two groups is that initiator caspases are active during the early, or reversible, stages of the apoptosis cascade, whereas activation of the so-called effector caspases is a subsequent transition that will ultimately lead to apoptotic cell death. The placental apoptosis cascade can be divided into three sets of sequential stages: i) *Initiation stages,* which include the induction of the cascade, e.g., by ligand-receptor interactions leading to first proteolytic events; ii) *Execution stages,* which start with the activation of the execution caspases. Their activation is called the 'point of no return' since once activated, these proteases degrade a variety of proteins resulting in irreversible damage of the cell; and iii) *Apoptotic death,* which is the result of a very complex cascade of events that finally leads to the collapse of the nucleus and the cell itself (Huppertz et al., 1999). Even at this final stage, the cell does not release intracellular components, thus avoiding inflammatory reactions (Huppertz et al., 1999).

Caspases are synthesized as inactive enzymes that require cleavage to exert their biologic roles. Initiator caspases 8 and 10 are activated in a subset of differentiated cytotrophoblasts, presumably destined for syncytial fusion (Huppertz et al., 2006). By contrast, effector caspases (3, 6, and 7) are expressed only in their inactive forms in the cytotrophoblast layer (Burton et al., 2003). Activation of the initiator caspase 8 is achieved by ligand-receptor interactions, eg, interactions between tumor necrosis factor- α (TNF- α) and the TNF-receptor 1 (TNF-R1) (Yui et al., 1996; Huppertz et al., 1998). The crucial role of caspase 8 in preparing cytotrophoblasts for syncytial fusion was demonstrated by Black et al., (2004). The activity of this caspase results in the cleavage of proteins linking the cytoskeleton to the plasma membrane, such as alpha-fodrin, and in the externalization of phosphatidylserine from the inner to the outer leaflet of the plasma membrane, a prerequisite for syncytial fusion. This is known to be a very early event during the initiation stages of apoptosis (Martin et al., 1995). Externalization of phosphatidylserine is used as a cellular signalling for events such as the attraction of macrophages, induction of the coagulation cascade or induction of syncytial fusion (Huppertz et al., 1999). Subsequently, initiator caspases cleave and activate a second subpopulation of caspases known as the execution caspases. Irreversible progression of the apoptosis cascade commences with activation of the latter. Execution caspase activation is tightly regulated by the bcl-2 family of mitochondrial proteins. The various members of this family promote or inhibit cleavage of execution caspases (Hockenberry et al., 1990).

It has been well established that, in general, once a cell has activated the effector caspase pathway, it will die by apoptosis within 24 hours. However, in the villous trophoblast, cytotrophoblast nuclei that enter the syncytiotrophoblast remain intact and viable for a few weeks. Once activated, the execution caspases, either directly or by means of other proteases, cleave a broad array of proteins critical for cell survival. The latter include intermediate filament proteins such as Cytokeratin 18 (Caulin et al., 1997), nuclear envelope proteins such as laminin A and B (Greidinger et al., 1996), DNA fragmentation factor (DFF) and other endonucleases, resulting in specific fragmentation of DNA (Liu et al., 1997). It has been shown that cytokeratin 18, which is cleaved by caspase 3 or 7, is affected in the early stages of apoptosis (Leers et al., 1999). The maintenance of trophoblast structure and its specialized function is essential for the provision of adequate oxygen levels and nutrients supply to the foetus. Apoptosis has been observed to naturally occur in placentas of normal human pregnancies, but as expected, placentas from women with PE or IUGR show enhanced apoptosis as compared to placentas of normal pregnant women (Allaire et al., 2000). The typical morphological signs of apoptosis (cellular shrinkage, membrane blebbing, nuclear condensation and fragmentation) are the final results of a complex biochemical cascade of events. The molecular mechanisms leading to apoptosis are complex, and include an ever-expanding list of signalling molecules such as the bcl-2 family of genes, the caspase-3 and NFκB (Hetts, 1998).

FETAL DEVELOPMENT AND OXIDATIVE STRESS

Exposure of the developing placenta, embryo or foetus to environmental agents like alcohol or acetaldehyde is known to produce anatomical anomalies leading to *in utero* death or structural birth defects (Gundogan et al., 2008), a process commonly termed teratogenesis (Wells et al,, 2009). The cellular mechanisms by which ethanol induce damage *in utero* are not yet well understood, although induction of oxidative stress is believed to be a putative mechanism due to an imbalance in prooxidant and antioxidant levels (Cohen-Kerem and Koren, 2003). Ethanol can induce oxidative stress directly and indirectly. The direct effect is achieved by the formation of free radicals, including hydroxyl and hydroxyethyl groups, which react with various cellular components. Formation of free radicals in the presence of ethanol was demonstrated in cell lines such as rat hepatocytes (Henderson et al,, 1995) as well as in the animal (Reinke et al,, 1987). The cellular damage caused by the presence of free radicals is a consequence of the peroxidation of lipids, nucleic acids and alterations of enzyme activity (Rodrigo et al., 2005). Another direct oxidative stress effect of ethanol is the formation of ROS (Dong et al., 2010), which are formed as biological products of molecular oxygen reduction (Fridovich, 1978) and they probably play a role in mediating programmed cell death (Jacobson, 1996; Dong et al., 2010).

The formation of ROS induced by cytochrome P-450 2E1 (CYP2E1) is mostly observed in the brain (Montoliu et al., 1995) and the liver (Morimoto et al., 1994), organs in which the enzyme is abundant. Formation of ROS is also induced by mitochondria in hepatocytes exposed to ethanol and is probably achieved by reduction in mitochondria-derived components of electron transport (Bailey and Cunningham, 1998).

Oxidative stress mechanism seems to operate in diabetes-induced embryonic damage as well as in the mechanism of teratogenicity caused by hypoxia and alcohol abuse (Ornoy, 2007). In addition, abnormal placentation may also cause enhanced placental oxidative stress, resulting in embryonic death, PE or congenital anomalies (Ornoy, 2007). Ethanol can also induce oxidative stress indirectly by reducing the intracellular antioxidant capacity, such as the levels of glutathione peroxidase. In rats, chronic ethanol consumption decreased significantly the cytosolic and mitochondrial glutathione peroxidase activities by 40% and 30%, respectively, and caused a parallel increase of the oxidative modification of proteins in hepatocytes (Oh et al., 1998; Bailey et al., 2001). The reason for the reduced activity of glutathione peroxidase might lie in the decreased mitochondrial pool size of glutathione because entry of cytosolic glutathione into mitochondria is impaired (Fernandez-Checa, 1991).

Enhanced production of ROS has also been suggested to be involved in the teratogenic process of ethanol-exposed pregnancy in experimental animals (Kotch et al., 1995; Chen and Sulik, 1996; Henderson et al., 1999) and pregnant women (Kay et al., 2000). Developing embryos seem to be very sensitive to high levels of ROS, especially during early organogenesis. High levels of oxygen are toxic to the embryo and foetus, apparently due to the fact that ROS created in such a condition are in excess in relation to the antioxidant capacity of the developing embryos, leading to the production of highly reactive oxygen or nitrogen species and creating oxidative/nitrative stress and embryonic damage, (Ornoy, 2007).

The effects of ROS and oxidative stress on placental, embryonic and fetal development may adversely alter the development by oxidative damage on the cellular lipids, proteins and DNA, and/or by altering signal transduction. Dysregulation of signal tranduction and/or macromolecular lesions can adversely alter cellular function or trigger apoptotic or necrotic cellular death (Wells et al., 2009). ROS such as hydrogen peroxide and hydroxyl radicals are formed via a variety of physiological and pathophysiological reactions, and ROS formation can be enhanced by xenobiotics (Fantel, 1996). To prevent free radical-induced cellular damage, the organism has developed a defence mechanism, the antioxidant system which includes antioxidant enzymes such as SOD, catalase (CAT), glutathione peroxidase (GSHPx), and glutathione reductase (GSSGR) and low molecular antioxidants such as glutathione and plasma proteins (Rodrigo et al, 2005). Although the levels of most antioxidative enzymes, with the exception of glucose-6-phosphate dehydrogenase (G6PD), are low in the embryo, there is some evidence that they nevertheless may provide protection against at least constitutive or physiological levels of ROS, if not drug-enhanced ROS formation (Wells et al., 2009). In addition to these, Henderson et al (1999) observed that ethanol induced oxidative stress in cultured fetal rat hepatocytes. The authors found that the supplementation with antioxidants or agents that enhance glutathione stores was able to reverse these effects.

The oxidative stress is associated with morphological and biochemical signs of mitochondrial damage. Ethanol inhibits activities of the mitochondrial respiratory chain components, a source that increased hydrogen peroxide, hydroxyl radicals, and lipid peroxidation products, along with signs of membrane damage. Additionally, the low antioxidant defences in fetal tissues and accumulation of toxic aldehyde products of lipid peroxidation predispose the foetus to oxidative damage. Wentzel et al. (2006) found that vitamin E treatment of pregnant chronic ethanol consuming rats diminishes fetal malformations. This study was in agreement with the study of Heaton et al., (2000), who blocked the effects of ethanol on Purkinje cells with the use of a very high dose of vitamin E. It seems likely that vitamins C and E could exert a protective effect by the reinforcement of antioxidant defences. An *in vitro* study reported evidence that vitamins C and E protect the strength and integrity of the chorioamnion from ROS-induced damage (Plessinger et al., 2000). However, some authors have not found a clear effect of antioxidant vitamin E supplementation (Tran et al., 2005), thereby raising the issue of the importance of dosage and variable sensitivity in different tissues towards both the deleterious effects of ethanol, as well as the beneficial effects of antioxidant vitamin E administration.

Henderson et al., (1999) found that supplementation with antioxidants or agents that enhance glutathione stores reversed the oxidative stress induced by ethanol in cultured fetal rat hepatocytes. In addition, Wentzel and Ekiksson (2008) demonstrated in rat embryos at 9-11 days of gestation, from 2 different rat strains exposed to 48 hours ethanol in early pregnancy, a role for genetic predisposition, oxidative stress, and apoptosis in ethanol teratogenicity, suggesting that the teratogenic predisposition of the more susceptible rat strain may reside, at least in part, in the regulation of the ROS scavenging enzymes. Folic acid acts also as an antioxidant, and Cano et al., (2001) studied its effects on oxidative stress induced by ethanol. Two groups of pregnant rats were chronically fed with ethanol-supplemented tap water up to a mean of 8.9 ± 0.4g ethanol/kg/day for 3 weeks. Reduction in glutathione reductase was significant in the group that received the high dosage of folic acid. The amount of carbonyl group proteins in the liver and pancreas was also used as an index for oxidative damage. Levels of carbonyl groups were reduced significantly in the liver of offspring supplemented with folic acid, but were unchanged in their pancreas. This study in an animal model showed an association between FAS and oxidative stress measurements and mitigation of those measures by using an antioxidant (Oh et al., 1998; Bailey et al., 2001). In addition, the study of Nasser et al. (2010) suggested that the antioxidant vitamin C could effectively reduce the severity of ethanol-induced brain injury and growth retardation by the modulation of γ-Aminobutiric acid receptor B (GABA$_B$ R) and protein kinase A-α (PKA) expression during early rat fetal development. Finally, Aliyu et al. (2009) evaluate whether the effect of alcohol use in SGA pregnacy is modified by maternal smoking behavior using a large database of linked birth registry records. The authors found that babies born to mothers with self-reported history of alcohol abuse during pregnancy had an increased risk of SGA and that this effect was enhanced by concomitant history of cigarette smoking.

ALCOHOL AND HYPERTENSION IN PREGNANCY

It has been demonstrated that pregnancy-induced hypertension contribute to low birth weight and preterm delivery (Bosco and Díaz, 2012). Although alcohol-associated hypertension is common among women who drink heavily (Asherio, et al., 1996; Seppa, et al., 1996), the effect of alcohol abuse on the course of hypertensive pregnancies has not been sufficiently studied. Mankes, et al., (1985) showed that alcohol administration during pregnancy increased hypertension, caused multiple birth defects, and increased fetal mortality in both normotensive and spontaneously hypertensive rats. In addition, Taylor et al. (1994) found that ethanol in the isolated perfused human placental lobule may contribute to the pathogenesis of the FAS as well as represent an underlying mechanism of ethanol-induced hypertension.

PE is a serius pregnancy complication, affecting 5-7% of all pregnancies, and is a leading cause of maternal and perinatal mortality. The placenta plays a pivotal role in the etiology of PE, specially the trophoblast cells of the placenta. PE is a two stage diseases which in the first stage, a reduction in uteroplacental perfusion and placental ischemia/hypoxia is caused by defective implantation and placentation. Placental hypoxia, in turn, may promote the release of a variety of factors to the maternal blood circulation, triggering the second stage, in which these factors initiate a cascade of cellular and molecular events leading to endothelial and vascular dysfunction (Caniggia et al., 2000). The latter leads to the maternal symptoms of the syndrome: hypertension, proteinuria and edema, which resolve spontaneously on placental delivery. Fetal complications of PE and IUGR are commonly attributed to clinical conditions that lead to a decrease in placental reperfusion, resulting in placental hypoxia (Levy et al., 2002). The pathogenic mechanisms of PE result in numerous stimuli, including oxidative stress, that lead finally to the endothelium dysfunction (Aban et al., 2004).

IMPAIRED PLACENTATION IN RAT FETAL ALCOHOL SYNDROME

Although IUGR is a key feature of FAS, its pathogenesis is still under investigation. Recently, Gundogan et al. (2008; 2010) demonstrated that chronic gestational exposure to ethanol in the rat causes increased fetal resorption as well as impairment in placental development and placentation. Since ethanol in maternal blood reaches the foetus and/or the placenta, its toxic effects on the foetus can be directly or indirectly mediated. The direct effect of fetal exposure to ethanol was demonstrated by Chu et al (2007) on rat fetal brain development and the indirect effect is related to placental pathology, especially within the labyrinthine rat placental barrier. The ischemia or infarction observed in ethanol–exposed placentas reduced thickness of the placenta by an increase in cellular necrosis. Since the exchange of nutrients between the mother and the foetus occurs within the labyrinthine layer, ethanol induced reductions in the mass of this layer could impair the delivery of nutrients to the rat foetus and thereby resulting in IUGR.

Gundogan et al. (2008; 2010) described that a second major placental abnormality associated with chronic gestational exposure to ethanol was failure of maternal uterine spiral arteries to remodelling from small muscular arteries to thin-walled, distended, flaccid vessels in order to produce the high-flow, low resistance circulation characteristic of intervillous space. Failure on maternal remodelling of uterine spiral arteries compromises both placental blood flow as well as the nutrients exchange (Pijnenborg et al., 1981b). Perturbation in this process has been linked to early pregnancy loss, IUGR and /or PE. Therefore, the motile and invasive properties of EVT are critical for establishing and maintaining pregnancy, and ensuring adequate blood and nutrient delivery to the foetus in order to support growth and development (Gundogan et al., 2008).

In addition, insulin-like growth factors (IGF) regulate placentation due to its stimulating effects on EVT, which are highly mobile and invasive (Gundogan et al., 2008). Previously, Gundogan et al. (2007) demonstrated that EVT express high levels of aspartyl-(asparaginyl) β-hydroxylase (AAH), a type 2 transmembrane protein with catalytic activity that hydroxylates epidermal growth factor-like domains of proteins that have a functional role in cell motility and invasion. AAH is regulated by IGF and has a critical role in cell motility and invasion, and recently, it has been demonstrated that ethanol impaired placentation is associated with inhibition of AAH expression in EVT (Gundogan et al., 2010).

HYPOXIC STRESS AND NEUROACTIVE STEROID RESPONSES

Compromised pregnancies can have serious effects on the fetal brain the nature of which depends, in large part, on the time of gestation they occur. Maternal stress, infections or problems with placentation can affect brain development due to changes in the delivery of oxygen and glucose to the brain, or the cytokine environment, leading to acute cell death (Hirst et al., 2009), particularly in vulnerable regions such as periventricular white matter, the hippocampus and the cerebellum (Inder et al., 1999; du Plessis and Volpe, 2002). It is also known that certain glial progenitor cells are highly susceptible to such insults. In addition, chronically suboptimal conditions during pregnancy dramatically increase the sensitivity of the fetal brain to further episodes of hypoxia/ischemia around the time of birth and in the immediate neonatal period. The resulting damage can lead to severe neuropathologies, including intellectual impairment and cerebral palsy (Inder et al., 1999).

The term neurosteroid has been used to refer to steroids synthesized *de novo* from cholesterol in the nervous system or, alternatively, when the last steps in synthesis take place in the nervous system. In pregnancy, a large proportion of the production of steroids that affect the fetal nervous system are derived from peripheral sources. Therefore, Hirst et al. (2009) used the term neuroactive steroids to refer to steroids that influence fetal or maternal nervous system function and may be synthesized both in the nervous system and/or other peripheral organs. Pregnancy is characterized by elevated neuroactive steroid levels both in the maternal circulation and brain, as well as in the fetal brain. The placenta is a source of considerable amounts of progesterone that enter not only into the maternal circulation, but also into the fetal blood and the fetal brain, where it is actively converted into the $GABA_A$ receptor active pregnane steroid, allopregnanolone (Crossley et al.,1997). Allopregnanolone is present in sufficient quantity to effectively raise the threshold for excitotoxicity in the fetal brain, as shown by the fact that severe fetal hypoxia produces greater damage when synthesis of allopregnanolone is suppressed (Yawno et al., 2007). More recent studies have suggested that progesterone metabolites may also have a role in development and repair of the fetal brain after exposure to hypoxia and other potential stressors in late pregnancy (Hirst et al., 2009). Evidence from animal studies indicates that elevated neuroactive steroid levels in pregnancy suppress excitability and increase lethargy (Paoletti et al., 2006). These results are consistent with the elevated plasma levels of $GABA_AR$ agonist steroids reported in women during pregnancy (Hill et al., 2007). These changes are resolved at birth with the removal of the placenta, suggesting that placental progesterone production is mostly responsible for the elevated neuroactive steroid levels in the plasma and their reported effects on mood (Gilbert Evans et al., 2005).

Disruption of placental function can cause chronic placental insufficiency and/or low placental perfusion, leading to IUGR. Although not always associated with marked pathology at birth, IUGR can cause severe or mild brain injury and it has been correlated with subtle developmental abnormalities evidenced later in life (Hirst et al., 2009). The impact of these complications on the developing brain is dependent upon the gestational age of the foetus at the time of injury and is also dependent on the time when the restriction becomes manifest (Inder and Volpe, 2000;

Frisk et al., 2002; Luciana, 2003). If placental function is reduced in early gestation, there is a concomitant reduction in body size. In contrast, limitation of placental function later in gestation results in asymmetrical growth restriction where the fetal head and brain are relatively less affected ('spared') compared to the body and somatic organs (Fang, 2005). In addition, progesterone has been found to act on gene expression in neural cells to promote myelination by interaction with associated Schwann cells. As progesterone receptors were not detectable in Schwann cells, these observations suggest a possible interaction between neuronal and glial cells in order to promote myelination (Schumacher et al., 2007).

It has been demonstrated that human and animals foetus prenatally exposed to alcohol have smaller brain size and thinner cerebral cortex, leading to significant decreases in the total cell number (Miller and Potempa, 1990; Miller, 1996; Ashwell and Zhang, 1996; Archibald et al., 2001). Amino acid-activated ion channels of excitatory (glutamate) and inhibitory (GABA) neurotransmitters in the prenatal rat brain have been shown to be altered in these foetuses (Lee et al., 1994; Allan et al., 1998; Nasser and Kim, 2010). Additionally, Ikonomidou, (2000) demonstrated that ethanol effects on the developing rat brain trigger a widespread neuronal death by blocking the N-methyl-D-aspartate (NMDA)–glutamate receptor and activating $GABA_A$ receptors. It has also been reported that neuroactive steroids reduce NMDA-induced excitotoxicity both *in vitro* (Lockhart et al., 2002) and *in vivo* models of brain injury (Djebaili et al., 2005). These excitatory pathways contribute to brain injury in the neonate following acute hypoxic episodes that may occur around the time of birth. In addition to being at risk of brain damage due to the chronic hypoxia alone, the IUGR foetus is also more susceptible to injury from acute hypoxia/ischemia-induced cell death at birth (Fang, 2005). Some studies show that greater damage is observed in vulnerable brain areas such as the hippocampus, brainstem and cortex, when asphyxia is sumperimposed on the already IUGR foetus. Burke et al. (2006) found that the dual insult of acute hypoxia in already IUGR foetuses resulted in a substantial potentiation of expression of apoptotic marker in the brain of neonatal piglets. Similarly, IUGR human neonates that were exposed to a period of asphyxia due to placental infarction showed increased brain injury (Burke and Gobe, 2005).

ALCOHOL-INDUCED NEURAL CREST CELLS APOPTOSIS

Exposure to alcohol consumption during gestation can have profound consequences, but not all cells within the embryo are equally affected. Studies in mice and chicks models have demonstrated that alcohol exposure at specific stages of early embryonic development results in significant death among cells destined to give rise to facial structures, as are the cranial neural crest cells (cNCC). Alcohol triggers apoptosis in retinoic acid (RA, a type of vitamin A) deficient cells from the neural crest, and also reduces levels of antioxidant compounds such as free radicals scavengers (Smith, 1997). Furthermore, Wentzel and Eriksson (2009), demonstrated on NCC of 10 day rat embryos that ethanol causes a shift towards apoptosis in both neural cells from cranial portion, and neural cells from trunk portion (tNCC), a shift which is diminished by treatment with the antioxidant N-acetylcysteine. Oxidative defense genes, and genes involved in NCC development are affected differently in cNCC compared to tNCC upon ethanol exposure. The cNCC Hox genes are downregulated, whereas tNCC are upregulated. These patterns of ethanol-altered gene expression may be of etiological importance for NCC-associated alterations of development in ethanol-exposed pregnancy.

Normal craniofacial morphology develops as a consequence of interactions between embryonic tissues such as cNCC, mesoderm and ectoderm, and requires precise regulation of cell movement, growth, patterning and differentiation of craniofacial tissue (Sant'Anna and Tosello, 2006). In addition, Oyedele and Cramer (2013) have demonstrated in avian cNCC how actin cytoskeleton (actin microfilament) disruption migratory distance, and proliferation are affected ex vivo by exposure to ethanol concentrations that simulate maternal intoxication. In mammalian embryos, the gastrulation period is characterized by intense mitotic activity, particularly in the developing mesoderm. Alcohol exposure during this period decrease the rate of cell division in mice embryos (C57B1/6J strain) (Sulikk, 1984), and the process of migration of mesodermal cells towards the primitive streak (Nakatsuji and Johnsson, 1984). Deficiencies in gastrulating mesodermal cells are responsible for inducing and maintaining neuroepithelial differentiation, an adverse effect on the mesoderm that could result in size reduction in the neural plate, which was particularly noticeable in the forebrain region (Sulikk et al., 1984).

Genetics studies have demonstrated the involvement of numerous genes in the craniofacial and dental structures, including genes encoding a variety of transcription factors, growth factors and receptors (Morris-Kay, 1993). The most common facial anomalies associated with FAS include short palpebral fissures, smooth philtrum, thin upper lip, midfacial hypoplasia and/or misaligned teeth (Jones et al., 1973). The craniofacial features include midfacial underdevelopment with gross shortage of bone, cranial base sloping to an extreme degree with backward-facing displacement of the cranio facial base, delayed dental development and enamel anomalies (Jackson and Hussain, 1990).

Although the cNCC contribute to form many tissues, alcohol-related research on these cells has been predominantly focused on facial bone and cartilage. Alcohol exposure cause cCNN apoptosis only if alcohol is administered before the CNN migrate from their birthplace into the neuroectoderm. Once the cells began the migration toward the site where the face will develops, CNN cells become resistant to alcohol-induced apoptosis (Cartwright and Smith, 1995). Studies in animal models have linked the characteristic facial abnormalities in FAS to cell death by apoptosis of cCNN during very well defined periods of vulnerability such as gastrulation or neurulation (Cartwright et al., 1998). One mechanism by which this may occurs is thought to be the formation of free radicals (Chen and Sulik, 1996). Others described mechanisms are deficiency in RA, altered expression of homeobox genes, intracellular communication and alterations in the activity of growth factors. All these mechanisms are likely interrelated, since RA is a key regulator of gene expression, and both free-radical toxicity and altered gene expression can produce apoptosis (Dickman et al., 1997; Smith, 1997).

The fact that alcohol also have an effect on odontogenesis make the tooth a good representative organ model to study developmental toxicity of ethanol (Kattainen et al., 2001). Bowden et al. (1983) have shown that ethanol exposure during pregnancy cause retardation of tooth eruption in offspring of macaque monkeys. Furthermore, Campos and Duranza (1988) found cellular alterations in the basal layer of the epithelium of the tooth germ in the bud stage and in the inner enamel epithelium in the mice.

Calmodulin Kinase II (CaMKII) is also affected by ethanol exposure. It has recently been shown in a chick embryo model that activated CaMKII was a novel and direct target of ethanol in neural cells progenitors. Ethanol exposure causes the rapid activation of CaMKII which is a molecular switch that converts calcium transient ethanol-activated into a regulator of survival and apoptosis of neural crest progenitor cells (Garic et al., 2011). Because neural crest cells differentiate into several neuronal lineages, these findings offer novel insights into how ethanol disrupts the processes of early neurogenesis. In addition, Zhou et al. (2011) found that alcohol exposure during the period of early neurulation is predominantly inhibitory to gene expression, particularly the neural developmental genes. These authors found major reductions in gene sets involved in neurospecification, neural growth factors, cell growth and hematopoiesis in mice embryos. Together, these genes should contribute to the generation of testable new hypotheses concerning the mechanistic pathway in gene expression changes leading to embryonic structural deficits, and for causal mechanisms of alcohol-induced teratogenesis (e.g., brain growth retardation, neural tube midline deficit, craniofacial dysmorphology) in the spectrum of fetal alcohol disorders.

ALTERATIONS IN BRAIN AND BEHAVIOUR BY FETAL ALCOHOL EXPOSURE

It is well known that heavy alcohol consumption throughout pregnancy leads to a significant risk of brain injury to the developing foetus, and that the latter is especially vulnerable to alcohol-induced brain injury during specific stages of brain development, many of which occur early during pregnancy (West, 1987; Ikonomidou et al., 2000). Thomas et al (2009) have shown in rats that Choline (an essential nutrient) supplementation during ethanol exposure significantly attenuated ethanol's effects on birth and brain weight, incisor emergence, and most behavioral measures. In fact, behavioral performance of ethanol-exposed subjects treated with choline did not differ from that of controls. Choline supplementation did not influence peak blood alcohol level or metabolism, indicating that choline's effects were not due to differential alcohol exposure. These data support the notion that early dietary supplements may reduce the severity of some fetal alcohol effects. In addition, Fukui and Fakata-Haga (2009), demonstrate in prenatal exposed ethanol rats, on the cerebral cortex, aberrant distribution of hippocampal mossy fibers and fussion of cerebelar folia. The authors concluded that the most certain way to prevent FAS/FASD is total abstinence during pregnancy and breastfeeding.

A recent work has demonstrated the neuroteratogenic effects of ethanol on *in vitro* human embryonic stem cells to neural human progenitors survival (Talens-Visconti et al, 2011). These authors found that ethanol exposure affects cell differentiation into neurons and astrocytes, disrupts the actin cytoskeleton, and affects expression of different genes associated with neural differentiation. Ethanol exposure during prenatal development causes a wide range of structural and functional brain abnormalities, affecting neurogenesis and gliogenesis, resulting in the FASD condition (Kumada et al., 2007). These authors summarised that the cellular mechanisms by which alcohol affects the migration of immature neurons are Ca^{+2} signalling and cyclic nucleotide signalling. Subtained exposure to alcohol during the period of gastrulation has a negative impact on the developing brain, reducing the neural cell progenitor pool (Rubert et al., 2006) and causing long-term effects on the forebrain (Ashwell and Zhang, 1996).

The cerebral cortex formation as well as the increase in both cortical surface area and neural cell number seems to be critical for the emergence of complex cognitive functions. The neural cell number is in turn dependent on the number of neural progenitor cells, their rate of proliferation and the mitotic cycles they undergo (Rubert et al., 2006). It has been reported that ethanol can induce microcephaly and deficits in cognitive functions and in some behavioral responses (Mattson and Riley, 1998). A critical period for ethanol induced microcephaly and teratogenesis has been shown to occurs during early embryogenesis in the rat brain, a period encompasing the first 10 day of gestation, equivalent to the first trimester in human (Maier et al., 1997; Guerri, 2002). During this period, the neural progenitor cells, radial glia (RG) are generated, and dysfunctions in its proliferation and survival could lead to an important reduction in the final number of neural cells.

In the development of the central nervous system (CNS) radial glia plays a role both as neural progenitors as well as scaffolding that supports neuronal migration Cameron and Rakic, 1994). The establishment of RG cells from the neuroepithelium precedes the generation and migration of neurons in the cerebral cortex. During early corticogenesis, RG cells generate neurons and then guide the daughter neurons in their ascent toward the developing cortical plate (Rakic, 1972; Komuro and Rakic, 1994,1998; Hatten, 1999). Once neuronal migration is completed, most RG disappear by differentiating into astrocytes (Rakic, 1995), the cells that play critical roles in the metabolic processes linked to neuronal activity such as blood flow, energy and glucose utilization (Magistretti, 2006). Recent findings have shown that RG cells are the predominant form of neural progenitors in the embryonic brain (Malatesta et al., 2000; Noctor et al., 2001; Gotz et al, 2005), giving rise to the majority of neurons in all CNS regions (Anthony et al., 2004). In addition, it has been recently suggested that the metabolic anomalies observed in different brain structures of individuals with FAS disorder are consistent with abnormalities in the glial cell pool, rather than in the neurons (Guerri et al, 2009, 2001).

The self-renewal capacity versus the specification of RG into the distinct neuronal and glial fates in the mammalian brain is regulated by intrinsic mechanisms, combined with extracellular temporal gradients of signalling molecules such as Notch (Rubert et al., 2006), and growth factors such as fibroblast growth factor 2 and epidermal growth factor (Temple, 2001). Hence, disruptions in these mechanisms and/or in the gradients of signalling molecules might affect neural progenitor cells and consequently CNS development. The study of Rubert et al. (2006) suggested that RG role as neuronal progenitor in the embryo may dramatically change the CNS development under normal and pathological conditions, such as those occurring during fetal alcohol exposure. It has also been found that pregnant rats chronically exposed to ethanol evidence inhibition of mitochondrial gene expression related with mitochondrial dysfunction, increased expression of pro-apoptotic and pro-oxidant genes with increased DNA damage and lipid peroxidation, and impaired insulin/insulin like growth factor signal transduction. Together, these results point to cerebellar hypoplasia (Chu et al, 2007).

A number of studies in animal models have provide evidence of the vulnerability of the CNS to the effects of ethanol, revealing that these effects are not uniform and that some brain areas or cell populations are more vulnerable than others (Guerri 1998; Guerri 2002; Tran and Kelly, 2003). Bonthius et al., (2008) found in cultured cerebellar granule cells from mouse pups that neuronal nitric oxide synthase (nNOS) protects developing neurons against alcohol toxicity by activating the nitric oxide and the cyclic GMP/ protein kinase G system on Ca^{2+} signalling and NFkappaB pathway. In addition, Kumar et al., (2010) demonstrated that high doses of ethanol affect the expression and activation of RA receptors, which could impair the signalling events and induce harmful effects on the survival and differentiation in rat cerebellar granule cells. In addition, the study of Rout and Dhossche (2010) showed that pregnant Long-Evans rats consumed significantly less of a protein fortified liquid-diet when the alcohol present in the diet is gradually increased and that the expression of molecules involved in the integrin signaling are significantly altered in the cerebral cortices of foetuses exposed to alcohol during gestation, even in the absence of obvious morphological defects in the offspring. Indeed, it has been well established that ethanol is a highly toxic substance for the developing fetal brain and, in fact, it is one of the leading preventable causes of birth defects and neurobehavioral disorders (American Academy of Pediatrics, 2000).

EFFECT OF ALCOHOL ON CARDIAC EMBRYO DEVELOPMENT

Cardiac malformations are frequently seen in FAS, the most common being ventricular septal defects (Sandor et al, 1981). Other associated anomalies are pulmonary artery hypoplasia and interruption of the aortic arch (Terrapon et al, 1977). Atrio-ventricular defects, patent ductus arteriosus and Fallot teratology have been observed to be associated with FAS (Loser et al, 1992). Recently, it has been found that exposure of zebrafish embryos to ethanol during development results in structural and functional changes in the heart that mimic malformations that occur in patients with FAS (Dlugos and Rabin, 2010).

In the previous paragraphs it has been described that alcohol alters the migration of neural crest cells. It is important to emphasises that in both avian and mammalian embryos a migration pathway is present from the occipital neural crest cells to the cardiac outflow tract, and that a disturbance in this area process can result in cardiac septation defects such as oartic pulmonary septum (Carlson, 2005), similar to that observed in cardiac malformations of FAS babies. Oxidative stress in the human placental villi induced by ethanol exposure may account for the decreased nitric oxide (NO) release, because NO may be shunted toward scavenging free radicals (Kay et al., 2000; Dotsch et al., 2001). In adition, Villamor et al., (2005) showed in chicken embryos that the chronic inhibition of NOS produced impairment of endothelium-dependent relaxation, structural remodeling of the pulmonary vascular bed and biventricular cardiac enlargement.

The ductus arteriosus (DA), a fetal arterial connection between the pulmonary artery and the descending aorta, is indispensable for fetal life. PGE 2 produces ductus relaxation by interacting with several of the PGE receptors (EP 2 , EP 3 , and EP 4). In the ductus, all three of the EP receptors participate in vasodilation by activating adenylate cyclase (Clymal, 2006). Following delivery there are several events that promote ductus constriction in the full term newborn: an increase in arterial PO 2 , a decrease in blood pressure within the ductus lumen (due to the postnatal decrease in pulmonary vascular resistance), a decrease in circulating PGE 2 (due to the loss of placental PG production and the increase in PG removal by the lung), and a decrease in the number of PGE 2 receptors in the ductus wall (Bouayad , 2001;Clymal, 2006). We postulate that the persistent of the ductus is probably due to the increased PGE2 concentration in the near-term foetus effects described by Brient and Smith (1991) in acute ethanol exposure on the near-term foetus. Vasodilator prostaglandins (PGs) appear to be the dominant vasodilators that oppose ductus constriction in the later part of gestation (Bouayad, 2001).

EFFECT OF ALCOHOL ON LIVER EMBRYO DEVELOPMENT

The liver is also affected in FAS and the characteristic deformities observed in this case are similar to those observed in alcoholic liver disease in adult. The features more commonly seen include hepatomegaly and raised serum transaminases. Light microscopy revealed increased parenchymal fat with portal and perisinusoidal spaces containing deposits of intermediated and large size collagen fibers, myo-fibroblast and occasional Ito cells, as well as subendothelial basement membrane-like material (Lefkowitch et al., 1983). The presence of thick sclerotic central veins in the liver lobule has also been evidenced, in conjunction with the occurrence of extrahepatic biliary atresia (Daft et al., 1986).

Furtheremore, Renau-Piqueras et al, (1997) demonstrated that prenatal exposure to ethanol affects the morphological, structural, and functional features of the Golgi apparatus, thus altering the glycosylation process in fetal hepatocytes, and producing accumulation of hepatic proteins. Additionally, Fofana et al., (2010), demonstrate that prenatal alcohol exposure alters phosphorylation of proteins in rat offspring liver and that the principal pathway affected by these protein alterations include cell signaling, cellular stress, protein synthesis, cytoskeleton, as well as glucose, aminoacid, adenosine and energy metabolism. Recently, Sozo et al (2013) demonstrated that daily ethanol exposure during the third-trimester-equivalent in sheep does not alter fetal liver morphology; however, decreased fetal liver ferric iron content and altered *hepcidin* and *ferroportin* gene expression indicate that iron homeostasis is indeed altered.

During pregnancy, there is coordinate expression of liver metallothionein (MT) (Zn-binding protein) in the mother and foetus. In the foetus, there is initially a very high level of MT expression in the placenta (early organogenesis), and then when the liver has developed and become functional there is a gradual increase in hepatic expression leading to parturition. Presumably, in the early stages, the placenta plays a major role in directing and mediating fetal zinc (Zn) homeostasis, and this role is gradually taken over by the fetal liver as it develops and becomes functional. It has been proposed that ethanol mediates significant changes in Zn homeostasis in the mother and foetus via induction of metallothionein (MT)-I and -II isoforms in the maternal liver (Carey et al, 2000). In addition, fetal Zn deficiency is one of the key mediators that underlie ethanol teratogenicity. There are remarkable similarities in fetal outcome between fetuses exposed to ethanol during development (Randall and Taylor, 1979; Sulik et al., 1981) and those that have endured a Zn-limiting environment through maternal insufficiency (Dreosti et al., 1986; Hurley et al., 1971).

EFFECT OF ALCOHOL ON LUNG EMBRYO DEVELOPMENT

In utero alcohol exposure dramatically increases the risk of premature delivery and understanding of the mechanisms of alcohol-induced alterations in the premature lung will advance the care of this vulnerable patient population. Therefore, given the various morbidities associated with prematurity, it is crucial to develop accurate and reliable methods for identifying alcohol exposed infants (Giliberti et al., 2013).

Fetal alcohol exposure promotes toxicity to developing organs, including the lung. At moderate levels, alcohol is primarily metabolized through alcohol dehydrogenase with class I and class IV alcohol dehydrogenase the primary isoforms in the developing lung (Ang et al., 1996). Since each polymorphism is associated with a different enzymatic activity, there will also be variances in alcohol metabolism within the developing lung (Gemma et al, 2007). Due to developing tissues such as the lung have poorly developed antioxidant systems, they are particularly vulnerable to alcohol induced oxidant stress and antioxidant depletion (Gautier et al., 2005; Sozo et al., 2009).

Additionally, it has been demonstrated that the innate immune response of lung epithelia represents the first line of defense against potentially pathogenic microorganisms present in inspired air. These responses can immediately prevent colonization and proliferation of microbes, thus minimizing the involvement of the adaptive immune response and allowing efficient gaseous exchange. Surfactant proteins A and D are additional components of pulmonary innate immunity and have an important role in pulmonary defense against inhaled pathogens (Lazic et al., 2007). Alveolar type II cells (ATII) as well as non-ciliated bronchial and bronchiolar epithelial cells (Clara cells) secrete lung surfactant. Surfactant is a mixture of phospholipids which primarily functions to prevent alveolar collapse during end-expiration (Ochs, 2006). Ethanol exposure significantly alters at least some of these lung innate responses (Lazic et al., 2007).

Multiple animal models of fetal alcohol exposure have demonstrated alterations in neonatal lung development. One mechanism for alcohol-induced impairment of lung rat development may be inhibition of glucose uptake or hormonal factors that regulate growth due to that fetal alcohol exposure decreases the release of insulin-like growth factor II (IGF-II) (Mauceri et la., 1994). In rats, fetal alcohol impairs lung development resulting in inhibition of cellular growth and hypoplastic lungs (Inselman et al., 1985) In mice, fetal alcohol during the second trimester at the pseudo glandular stage of lung development resulted in decreased lung mass and delayed lung maturation (Wang et al, 2007). These effects of *in utero* alcohol were also associated with increased expression of the homeobox-containing gene Hoxb5 which is critical for bronchiolar patterning and airway branching morphogenesis during the saccular phase of development. However, dramatic decreases in Hoxb5 expression are needed for bronchiole elongation and further lung development. Thus, persistent Hoxb5 expression further supports the concept that foetal alcohol exposure impairs lung development (Wang et al., 2007). In preterm lambs with fetal alcohol exposure during the last trimester of pregnancy, there was decreased expression of vascular endothelial growth factor (VEGF) which is critical for angiogenesis, endothelial cell maturation and alveolar formation (Lazic, 2011). Also, in utero alcohol exposure alters the developing immune system and decreases pulmonary defences against both bacterial and viral infection (Giliberti et al., 2013). Newborns have an increased baseline risk for pneumonia as many normal adult lung defences are compromised in the foetus and newborn including the ciliary escalator, airway macrophages and dendritic cells, secretory antibodies, and antimicrobial proteins and antigens (Nissen, 2007). Increased incidence of neonatal pneumonia is multifactorial; however, animal models show an increased risk for pneumonia in foetal alcohol exposure (Gauthier et al., 2009). Continued research is required to fully identify and understand the effects of in utero alcohol on infection risk and infectious-mediated pulmonary morbidities, particularly in at-risk premature newborn.

SUMMARY AND CONCLUSIONS

We have reviewed a number of published studies concerning the principal evidences of the teratogenic effects of prenatal ethanol exposure on placentation, placenta growth, placenta function, and fetal development with emphasis in the development of the central nervous system, heart, lung and liver. The focus of this review gives special relevance to the association between the teratogenic effect, hypoxia and oxidative stress, the molecular mechanism involved (e.g. apoptosis) and the range of effects. The studies in this field provide a comprehensive picture of the association among structural and functional placenta abnormalities and structural and functional brain, heart, lung and liver abnormalities, in order to identify factors that mediate the relationship between alcohol exposure during pregnancy and the risk of extreme premature delivery shown by individual with FAS/FASD.

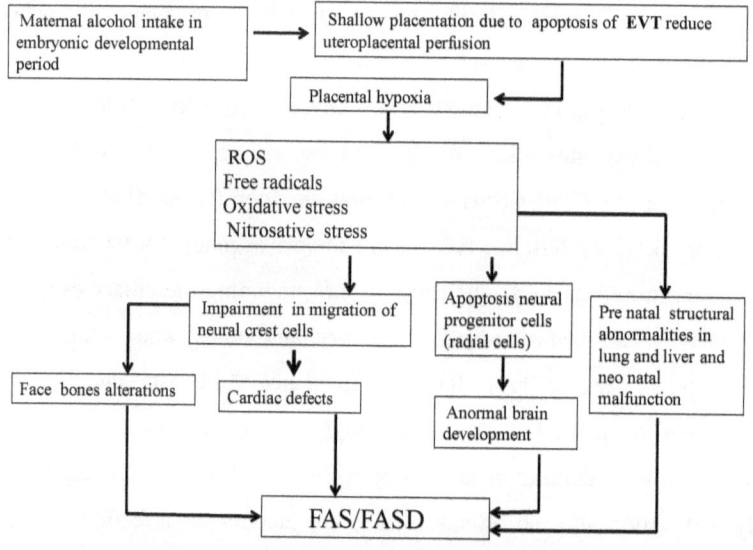

Figure 1: Model representation of the effect of maternal alcohol consumption on first stages of placental development. During the first weeks of gestation (weeks 10–12), placental development occurs in a normal hypoxic environment. Exposure to alcohol by maternal consumption during this period will trigger the hypoxic effect of alcohol or acetaldehyde, which in turn will increase the hypoxicity of the environment. As a result, hypoxia will be higher than normal and the response will depend on constitutional maternal factors, as well as on the ability of the placenta to react. If this hypoxic situation persists beyond weeks 10–12, the differentiation of CTF to ETV will decrease, producing a shallow placentation, in addition to a diminished uterine irrigation of the

organ. The latter will induce an oxidative stress in the placenta, altering consequently the normal embryo and/or fetal development, specially brain, face, heart, liver and lung.

Acknowledgments: This research was supported in part by Grant EDID 99009, from Departamento Técnico de Investigación y Desarrollo (DTI), Universidad de Chile.

REFERENCES

Aban M, Cinel L, Arslan M, Dilek U, Kapanoglu M, Arpaci R, Dilek S (2004) Expression of nuclear factor-kappa B and placental apoptosis in pregnancies complicated with intrauterine growth restriction and preeclampsia: an immunohistochemical study. *Tohoku Journal of Experimental Medicine* **204**, 195-202.

Aliyu M, Wilson R, Zoorob R, Brown K, Alio A, Clayton H, Salihu H. (2009) Prenatal alcohol consumption and fetal growth restriction: potentiation effect by concomitant smoking. *Nicotine & Tobacco Research* **11**, 36-43.

Allaire AD, Ballenger KA, Wells SR, McMahon MJ, Lessey BA (2000) Placental apoptosis in preeclampsia. *Obstetrics and Gynecology* **96**, 271-276.

Allan AM, Wu H, Paxton LL, Savage DD (1998) Prenatal ethanol exposure alters the modulation of the gamma-aminobutyric acid A1 receptor-gated chloride ion channel in adult rat offspring. *Journal of Pharmacology and Experimental Therapeutics* **284**, 250-257

American Academy of Pediatrics. Committee on Substance Abuse and Committee on Children with Disabilities (2000) Fetal Alcohol Syndrome and Alcohol-Related Neurodevelopmental Disorders. *Pediatrics* **106**, 358-361.

Ang HL, Deltour L, Zgombić-Knight M, Wagner MA, Duester G (1996) Expression patterns of class I and class IV alcohol dehydrogenase genes in developing epithelia suggest a role for alcohol dehydrogenase in local retinoic acid synthesis. *Alcoholism, Clinical and Experimental Research* **20(6)**, 1050-1064.

Anthony TE, Klein C, Fishell G, Heintz N (2004) Radial glia serves as neuronal progenitors in all regions of the central nervous system. *Neuron* **41**, 881-890.

Aplin JD (1991) Implantation, trophoblast differentiation and haemochorial placentation: mechanistic evidence in vivo and in vitro. *Journal of Cell Science* **99**, 681-692.

Archibald SL, Fennema-Notestine C, Gamst A, Riley EP, Mattson SN, Jernigan TL (2001) Brain dysmorphology in individuals with severe prenatal alcohol exposure. *Developmental Medicine and Child Neurology* **43**, 148-154.

Ascherio A, Hennekens C, Willett WC, Sacks F, Rosner B, Manson J, Witteman J, Stampfer M (1996) Prospective study of nutritional factors, blood pressure, and hypertension among US women. *Hypertension* **27**, 1065-1072.

Ashwell KW, Zhang LL (1996) Forebrain hypoplasia following acute prenatal ethanol exposure: quantitative analysis of effects on specific forebrain nuclei. *Pathology* **28**, 161-166

Baeuerle PA, Henkel T (1994) Function and activation of NF-kappa B in the immune system. *Annual Review of Immunology* **12**,141-79.

Bailey SM, Cunningham CC (1998) Acute and chronic ethanol increases reactive oxygen species generation and decreases viability in fresh, isolated rat hepatocytes. *Hepatology* **28**, 1318-1326.

Bailey SM, Patel VB, Young TA, Asayama K, Cunningham CC (2001) Chronic ethanol consumption alters the glutathione/glutathione peroxidase- 1 system and protein oxidation status in rat liver. *Alcoholism, Clinical and Experimental Research* **25**, 726-733.

Baldwin AS Jr (1996) The NF-kappa B and I kappa B proteins: new discoveries and insights. *Annual Review of Immunology*. **14**, 649-83

Banan A, Fields JZ, Decker H, Zhang Y, Keshavarzian A (2000) Nitric oxide and its metabolites mediate ethanol-induced microtubule disruption and intestinal barrier dysfunction. *Journal of Pharmacology and Experimental Therapeutics* **294**, 997-1008.

Banan A, Fields JZ, Zhang Y, Keshavarzian A (2001) iNOS upregulation mediates oxidant-induced disruption of F-actin and barrier of intestinal monolayers. *American Journal of Physiology. Gastrointestinal and Liver Physiology* **280**, G1234-G1246.

Beckman JS, Ye YZ, Anderson PG, Chen J, Accavitti MA, Tarpey MM, White CR (1994) Extensive nitration of protein tyrosines in human atherosclerosis detected by immunohistochemistry. *Biological Chemistry Hoppe Seyler* **375**, 81-88.

Black S, Kadyrov M, Kaufmann P, Ugele B, Emans N, Huppertz B (2004) Syncytial fusion of human trophoblast depends on caspase 8. *Cell Death and Differentiation* **11**, 90-98.

Bonfoco E, Krainc D, Ankarcrona M, Nicotera P, Lipton SA (1995) Apoptosis and necrosis: two distinct events induced, respectively, by mild and intense insults with *N*-methyl-D-aspartate or nitric oxide/superoxide in cortical cell cultures. *Proceedings of the National Academy of Sciences of the United States of America* **92**, 7162-7166.

Bonizzi G, Karin M (2004) The two NF-kappaB activation pathways and their role in innate and adaptive immunity. *Trends in Immunology* **25**, 280-288.

Bonthius DJ, Bonthius NE, Karacay B (2008) The protective effect of neuronal nitric oxide synthase (nNOS) against alcohol toxicity depends upon NO-cGMP-PKG pathway and NF-kappaB. *Neurotoxicology* **29**, 1080-1091.

Bosco C (1994) Morphology of the capillaries in the alpha and beta zone of human term placenta: the relationship between capillary morphology and the trophoblastic layer. *Medical Science Research* **22**, 115-117.

Bosco C (1995) The cytotrophoblast: The first human amine precursor uptake and decarboxylation (APUD) cell. *Medical Science Research* **23**, 205-207

Bosco C. (2005) Alcohol and Xenobiotics in Placenta Damage. In Preedy, V.R and Watson, R.R (eds) *Comprehensive Handbook of Alcohol Related Pathology*, Vol.2, pp 921-935. London: Elsevier Science.

Bosco C, Díaz E (2012) Placental hypoxia and foetal development versus alcohol exposure in pregnancy. *Alcohol and Alcoholism* **47(2)**, 109-117.

Bosco C, González J, Gutiérrez R, Parra-Cordero M, Barja P, Rodrigo R (2012) Oxidative damage to pre-eclamptic placenta: immunohistochemical expression of VEGF, nitrotyrosine residues and von Willebrand factor. *Journal of Maternal and Fetal Neonatal Medicine* **25**, 2339-2345.

Bouayad A, Kajino H, Waleh N, Fouron JC, Andelfinger G, Varma DR, Skoll A, Vazquez A, Gobeil F Jr, Clyman RI, Chemtob S (2001) Characterization of PGE 2 receptors in fetal and newborn lamb ductus arteriosus. *American Journal of Physiology* **280**, H2342–H2349.

Bowden DM, Weathersbee PS, Clarren SK, Fahrenbruch CE, Goodlin BL, Caffery SA (1983) A periodic dosing model of fetal alcohol syndrome in the pig-tailed macaque (Macaca nemestrina). *American Journal of Primatology* **4**, 143-157.

Brien JF, Chan D, Green CR, Iqbal U, Gareri J, Kobus SM, McLaughlin BE, Klein J, Rao C, Reynolds JN, Bocking AD, Koren G (2006) Chronic prenatal ethanol exposure and increased concentration of fatty acid ethyl esters in meconium of term fetal Guinea pig. *Therapeutic Drug Monitoring* **28**, 345-350.

Brien JF, Smith GN (1991) Effects of alcohol (ethanol) on the fetus. *Journal of Developmental Physiology* **15**, 21-32.

Brookes PS (2004) Mitochondrial nitric oxide synthase. *Mitochondrion* **3**,187-204.

Brown GC, Borutaite V (1999) Nitric oxide, cytochrome *c* and mitochondria. *Biochemical Society Symposium* **66**, 17-25.

Burke C, Gobe G (2005) Pontosubicular apoptosis ('necrosis') in human neonates with intrauterine growth retardation and placental infarction. *Virchows Archiv: an International Journal of Pathology* **446**, 640-645.

Burke C, Sinclair K, Cowin G, Rose S, Pat B, Gobe G, Colditz P (2006) Intrauterine growth restriction due to uteroplacental vascular insufficiency leads to increased hypoxia- induced cerebral apoptosis in newborn piglets. *Brain Research* **1098**, 19-25.

Burner U, Furtmüller PG, Kettle AJ, Koppenol WH, Obinger C (2000) Mechanism of reaction of myeloperoxidase with nitrite. *The Journal of Biological Chemistry* **275**, 20597-20601.

Burney S, Caulfield JL, Niles JC, Wishnok JS, Tannenbaum SR (1999) The chemistry of DNA damage from nitric oxide and peroxynitrite. *Mutation Research* **424**, 37-49.

Burton G L, Skepper JN, Hempstock J, Cindrova T, Jones CJ, Jauniaux E (2003) A reppraisal of the contrasting morphological appearances of villous cytotrophoblast cells during early human pregnancy; evidence for both apoptosis and primary necrosis. *Placenta* **24**, 297-305.

Cameron RS, Rakic P (1994) Identification of membrane proteins that comprise the plasmalemmal junction between migrating neurons and radial glial cells. *Journal of Neuroscience* **14**, 3139-3155.

Campos RM, Duranza MC (1988) Efectos del consumo prolongado de etanol sobre las etapas tempranas del desarrollo dentario en ratones. *Revista Cubana de Investigaciones Biomédicas* **7**, 30-35.

Caniggia I., Winter J, Lye SJ, Post M (2000) Oxygen and placental development during the first trimester : implications for the pathophysiology of pre-eclampsia. *Placenta* **21**, S25-S30.

Cano MJ, Ayala A, Murillo ML, Carreras O (2001) Protective effect of folic acid against oxidative stress produced in 21-day postpartum rats by maternal-ethanol chronic consumption during pregnancy and lactation period. *Free Radical Research* **34**, 1-8.

Caulin C, Salvesen GS, Oshima RG (1997) Caspase cleavage of keratin 18 and reorganization of intermediate filaments during epithelial cell apoptosis. *Journal of Cell Biology* **138**, 1379-1394.

Carey LC, Coyle P,. Philcox JC, Rofe AM. (2000) Ethanol Decreases Zinc Transfer to the Fetus in Normal but Not Metallothionein-Null Mice. *Alcoholism: Clinical and Experimental Research.* **24**, 1236–1240.

Carlson B (2005) Células de la cresta neural. In Carlson B (ed). *Embriología Humana y Biología del Desarrollo*, pp 277-290. Spain Elsevier Science.

Cartwright MM, Smith SM (1995) Increased cell death and reduced neural crest cell numbers in ethanol-exposed embryos: partial basis for the fetal alcohol syndrome phenotype. *Alcoholism, Clinical and Experimental Research* **19**, 378-386.

Cartwright MM, Tessmer LL, Smith SM (1998) Ethanol induced neural crest apoptosis is coincident with their endogenous death, but is mechanistically distinct. *Alcoholism, Clinical and Experimental Research* **22**, 142-149.

Chan D, Klein J, Karaskov T, Koren G (2004) Fetal exposure to alcohol as evidence by fatty acid ethyl esters in meconium in the absence of maternal drinking history in pregnancy. *Therapeutic Drug Monitoring* **26**, 474-481.

Chang W, Webster DR, Salam AA, Gruber D, Prasad A, Eiserich JP, Bulinski JC (2002) Alteration of the C-terminal amino acid of tubulin specifically inhibits myogenic differentiation. *Journal of Biological Chemistry* **277**, 30690-30698.

Chaudhuri J (2000) Alcohol and the developing fetus- a review. *Medical Science Monitor* **6**, 1031-1041.

Chen S, Sulik KK (1996) Free radicals and ethanol-induced cytotoxicity in neural crest. *Alcoholism, Clinical and Experimental Research* **20**, 1071-1076.

Chen LW, Egan L, Li ZW, Greten FR, Kagnoff MF, Karin M (2003) The two faces of IKK and NF-kappaB inhibition: prevention of systemic inflammation but increased local injury following intestinal ischemia-reperfusion. *Nature Medicine* **9**, 575-581.

Chesnutt C, Burrus LW, Brown AM, Niswander L (2004) Coordinate regulation of neural tube patterning and proliferation by TGFbeta and WNT activity. *Developmental Biology* **274**, 334–347.

Chu J, Tong M, de la Monte SM (2007) Chronic ethanol exposure causes mitochondrial dysfunction and oxidative stress in immature central nervous system neurons. *Acta Neuropathologica* **113**, 659-673.

Chudley AE, Conry J, Cook JL, Look C, Rosales T, LeBlanc N (2005) Fetal alcohol spectrum disorder: Canadian guidelines for diagnosis. *Canadian Medical Association Journal*, **172**, S1–S21.

Clements MK, Siemsen DW, Swain SD, Hanson AJ, Nelson-Overton LK, Rohn TT, Quinn MT (2003). Inhibition of actin polymerization by peroxynitrite modulates neutrophil functional responses. *Journal of Leukocyte Biology* **73**, 344-355.

Cohen-Kerem R, Koren G (2003) Antioxidants and fetal protection against ethanol teratogenicity I. Review of the experimental data and implications to humans. *Neurotoxicology and Teratology* **25**, 1-9.

Cooke CL, Davidge ST (2002) Peroxynitrite increases iNOS through NF-κB and decreases prostacyclin synthase in endothelial cells. *American Journal of Physiology. Cell Physiology* **282**, C395-C402.

Crocker IP, Cooper S, Ong SC, Baker PN (2003) Differences in apoptotic susceptibility of cytotrophoblasts and syncytiotrophoblasts in normal pregnancy to those complicated with preeclampsia and intrauterine growth restriction. *American Journal of Pathology* **162**, 637-643.

Cross CJ (2006) Placental function in development and disease. *Reproduction, Fertility and Development* **18**, 71-76.

Cross CJ, Werb Z, Fisher SJ (1994) Implantation and the placenta: key pieces of the development puzzle. *Science* **26**, 1508-1517.

Crossley KJ, Nicol MB, Hirst JJ, Walker DW, Thorburn GD (1997) Suppression of arousal by progesterone in fetal sheep. *Reproduction, Fertility, and Development* **9**, 767-773.

Clyman RI (2006) Mechanisms regulating the ductus arteriosus. *Biology of the Neonate* **89**, 330–335.

Daft PA, Johnston MC, Sulik KK (1986) Abnormal heart and great vessel development following acute ethanol exposure in mice. *Teratology* **33**, 93-104.

Delaval K, Feil R (2004) Epigenetic regulation of mammalian genomic imprinting. *Current Opinion in Genetics & Development* **14**, 188–195.

Denicola A, Radi R (2005) Peroxynitrite and drug-dependent toxicity. *Toxicology* **15**, 273-288.

Djebaili M, Guo Q, Pettus EH, Hoffman SW, Stein DG (2005) The neurosteroids progesterone and allopregnanolone reduce cell death, gliosis, and functional deficits after traumatic brain injury in rats. *Journal of Neurotrauma* **22**, 106-118.

Dickhout JG, Hossain GS, Pozza LM, Zhou J, Lhotak S, Austin RC (2005) Peroxynitrite causes endoplasmic reticulum stress and apoptosis in human vascular endothelium: implications in atherogenesis. *Arteriosclerosis, Tthrombosis, and Vascular Biology* **25**, 2623-2629.

Dickman S (1997) Possible new roles for HOX genes. *Science* **278 (5345)**, 1882-1883.

Dlugos CA, Rabin RA (2010) Structural and functional effects of developmental exposure to etanol on the zebrafish Heart. *Alcoholism, Clinical and Experimental Research* **34**, 1-9.

Dong J, Sulik KK, Chen SY (2010) The role of NOX enzymes in ethanol-induced oxidative stress and apoptosis in mouse embryos. *Toxicology Letters* **193**, 94-100.

Dotsch J, Hogen N, Nyul Z, Hanze J, Knerr I, Kirschbaum M, Rascher W (2001). Increase of endothelial nitric oxide synthase and endothelin-1 mRNA expression in human placenta during gestation. *European Journal of Obstetrics & Gynecology and Reproductive Biology* **97**, 163-167.

Dreosti IE, Buckley RA, Chem HCA, Record IR (1986) The teratogenic effect of zinc deficiency and accompanying feeding patterns in mice. *Nutrition Research* **6**, 159-166.

du Plessis AJ, Volpe JJ (2002) Perinatal brain injury in the preterm and term newborn. *Current Opinion in Neurology* **15**, 151-157.

Enders AC (1965) A comparative study of the fine structure of the trophoblast in several hemochorial placentas. *American Journal of Anatomy* **116**, 29-67.

Fang S (2005) Management of preterm infants with intrauterine growth restriction. *Early Human Development* **81**, 889-900.

Fantel AG (1996) Reactive oxygen species in developmental toxicity: review and hypothesis. *Teratology* **53**, 196-217

Fernandez-Checa JC, Garcia-Ruiz C, Ookhtens M, Kaplowitz N (1991) Impaired uptake of glutathione by hepatic mitochondria from chronic ethanol-fed rats. Tracer kinetic studies in vitro and in vivo and susceptibility to oxidant stress. *Journal of Clinical Investigation* **87**, 397-405.

Fisher SE, Atkinson M, Burnap JK, Jacobson S, Sehgal PK, Scott W, Van Thiel DH (1982) Ethanol-associated selective fetal malnutrition: a contributing factor in the fetal alcohol syndrome. *Alcoholism, Clinical and Experimental Research* **6**, 197-201.

Fisher SE, Karl PI (1988) Maternal ethanol use and selective fetal malnutrition. *Recent Development in Alcoholism* **6**, 277-289.

Fridovich I (1978) The biology of oxygen radicals. *Science* **201**, 875-880.

Floris R, Piersma SR, Yang G, Jones P, Wever R (1993) Interaction of myeloperoxidase with peroxynitrite. A comparison with lactoperoxidase, horseradish peroxidase and catalase. *European Journal of Biochemistry* **215**, 767-775.

Floyd RL, Decofle P, Hungerfond DW (1999) Alcohol use prior to pregnancy recognition. *American Journal of Preventive Medicine* **12**, 101-107.

Floyd RL, Weber MK, Denny C, O´Connor MJ (2009) Prevention of fetal alcohol spectrum disorders. *Developmental Disabilities Research Reviews* **15**, 193-199.

Fofana B, Yao XH, Rampitsch C, Cloutier S, Wilkins JA, Nyomba BL (2010) Prenatal alcohol exposure alters phosphorylation of proteins in rat offspring liver. *Proteomics* **10**, 417-434

Frisk V, Amsel R, Whyte HE (2002) The importance of head growth patterns in predicting the cognitive abilities and literacy skills of small-for-gestational-age children. *Developmental Neuropsychology* **22**, 565–593.

Fukui Y, Sakata-Haga H (2009) Intrauterine invironment-genome interaction and Children´s development (1) : Ethanol a teratogen in developing brain. *The Journal of Toxicological Science* **34** (II), SP273-SP278.

Gahagan S, Sharpe TT Brimacombe M, Fry-Johnson Y, Levine R, Mengel M, O'Connor M, Paley B (2006) Pediatricians' knowledge, training, and experience in the care of children with fetal alcohol syndrome. *Pediatrics* **118**, 657-658.

Gareri J, Brien J, Reynolds J, Koren G (2009) Potential role of the placenta in fetal alcohol spectrum disorder. *Paediatrics Drugs* **11**, 26-29.

Garic A, Flentke G, Amberger E, Hernandez M, Smith S (2011) CaMKII activation is a novel effector of alcohol´s neurotoxicity in neural crest stem/progenitor cells. *Journal of Neurochemistry* **118**, 646–657.

Gauthier TW, Ping XD, Harris FL, Wong M, Elbahesh H, Brown LA (2005) Fetal alcohol exposure impairs alveolar macrophage function via decreased glutathione availability. *Pediatric Research* **57(1)**, 76-81.

Gauthier TW, Young PA, Gabelaia L, Ping XD, Harris FL, Brown LA (2009) In utero ethanol exposure impairs defenses against experimental group B streptococcus in the term Guinea pig lung. *Alcoholism, Clinical and Experimental Research* **33**, 300–306.

Gemma S, Vichi S, Testai E (2007) Metabolic and genetic factors contributing to alcohol induced effects and fetal alcohol syndrome. *Neuroscience and Biobehavioral Reviews* **31**, 221–229.

Gemma S, Vichi S, Testai E (2006) Individual susceptibility and alcohol effects: biochemical and genetic aspects. *Annali dell'Istituto Superiore di Sanità* **42**, 8–16.

Genbacev O, Zhou Y, Ludlow J W, Fisher S J (1997). Regulation of human placental development by oxygen tension. *Science* **27**, 1669-1672.

Gilbert Evans SE, Ross LE, Sellers EM, Purdy RH, Romach MK (2005) 3 alpha-reduced neuroactive steroids and their precursors during pregnancy and the postpartum period. *Gynecological Endocrinology* **21**, 268–279.

Giles S, Boehm P, Brogan C, Bannigan J (2008) The effects of ethanol on CNS development in the chick embryo. *Reproductive Toxicology* **25**, 224–230.

Giliberti D, Mohan SS, Brown LA, Gauthier TW (2013) Perinatal exposure to alcohol: implications for lung development and disease. *Paediatric Respiratory Reviews* **14(1)**, 17-21.

Gotz M, Barde YA (2005) Radial glial cells defined and major intermediates between embryonic stem cells and CNS neurons. *Neuron* **46**, 369–372.

Greidinger EL, Miller DK, Yamin TT, Casciola-Rosen L, Rosen A (1996) Sequential activation of three distinct ICE-like activities in Fas-ligated Jurkat cells. *FEBS Letters* **390(3)**, 299-303.

Gu Y, Srivastava RK, Clarke DL, Linzer DI, Gibori G (1996) The decidual prolactin receptor and its regulation by decidua-derived factors. *Endocrinology* **137**, 4878-4885.

Guerri C (1998) Neuroanatomical and neurophysiological mechanisms involved in central nervous system dysfunctions induced by prenatal alcohol exposure. *Alcoholism, Clinical and Experimental Research* **22**, 304-312.

Guerri C, Pascual M, Renau-Piqueras J (2001). Glia and fetal alcohol syndrome. *Neurotoxicology* **22**, 593–599.

Guerri C (2002) Mechanisms involved in central nervous system dysfunctions induced by prenatal ethanol exposure. *Neurotoxicology Research* **4**, 327– 335.

Guerri C, Bazinet A, Riley EP (2009) Foetal alcohol spectrum disorders and alterations in brain and behaviour. *Alcohol & Alcoholism* **44**, 108-114.

Gundogan F, Elwood G, Greco D, Rubin LP, Pinar H, Carlson RI, Wands JR, de la Monte SM (2007) Role of aspartyl-(asparagyl) beta-hydroxylase in placental implantation : relevance to early pregnancy loss. *Human Pathology* **38**, 50-59.

Gundogan F, Elwood G, Longato L, Tong M, Feijoo A, Carlson RI, Wands JR, de la Monte SM (2008) Impaired placentation in fetal alcohol syndrome. *Placenta* **29**, 148-157.

Gundogan F, Elwood G, Mark P, Feijoo A, Longato L, Tong M, de la Monte SM (2010) Ethanol-induced oxidative stress and mitochondrial dysfunction in rat placenta: relevance to pregnancy loss. *Alcoholism, Clinical and Experimental Research* **34**, 415-423.

Hatten ME (1999) Central nervous system neuronal migration. *Annual Review of Neuroscience* **22**, 511-539.

Heasell AEP, Crocker IP (2008) Live and Let Die – Regulation of Villous Trophoblast Apoptosis in Normal and Abnormal Pregnancies. *Placenta* **29**, 772-783

Heaton MB, Mitchell JJ, Paiva M (2000) Amelioration of ethanol induced neurotoxicity in the neonatal rat central nervous system by antioxidant therapy. *Alcoholism, Clinical and Experimental Research* **24**, 512-518.

Henderson GI, Devi BG, Perez A, Schenker S (1995) In utero ethanol exposure elicits oxidative stress in the rat fetus. *Alcoholism, Clinical and Experimental Research* **19**, 714- 720.

Henderson GI, Chen JJ, Schenker S (1999) Ethanol, oxidative stress, reactive aldehydes, and the fetus. *Frontiers in Bioscience* **15**, D541-D550.

Hetts SW (1998) To die or not to die: an overview of apoptosis and its role in disease. *Journal of American Medical Association* **279**, 300-307.

Hill M, Cibula D, Havlíková H, Kancheva L, Fait T, Kancheva R, Parízek A, Stárka L (2007) Circulating levels of pregnanolone isomers during the third trimester of human pregnancy. *Journal of Steroid Biochemistry and Molecular Biology* **105**, 166-175

Hirst JJ, Walker DW, Yawno T, Palliser HK (2009) Stress in pregnancy: a role for neuroactive steroids in protecting the fetal and neonatal brain. *Developmental Neuroscience* **31**, 363-377.

Hockenberry D, Nunez G, Milliman C, Schreiber RD, Korsmeyer SJ (1990) Bcl-2 is an inner mitochondrial membrane protein that blocks programmed cell death. *Nature* **348**, 334-336.

Huppertz B, Kadyrov M, Kingdom JC (2006) Apoptosis and its role in the trophoblast. *American Journal of Obstetrics and Gynecology* **195**, 29-39.

Huppertz B, Frank HG, Kaufmann P (1999) The apoptosis cascade– morphological and immunohistochemical methods for its visualization. *Anatomy and Embryology* **200**, 1-18.

Huppertz B, Frank H G, Kingdom J C, Reister F, Kaufmann P (1998) Villous cytotrophoblast regulation of the syncytial apoptotic cascade in the human placenta. *Histochemistry and Cell Biology* **110**, 495-508.

Hurley LS, Gowan J, Swenerton H (1971) Teratogenic effects of short term and transitory zinc deficiency in rats. *Teratology* **4**, 199 –204.

Ikonomidou C, Bittigau P, Ishimaru MJ, Wozniak DF, Koch C, Genz K, Price MT, Stefovska V, Hörster F, Tenkova T, Dikranian K, Olney JW (2000) Ethanol-induced apoptotic neurodegeneration and fetal alcohol syndrome. *Science* **287**, 1056-1060.

Inder TE, Volpe JJ (2000) Mechanisms of perinatal brain injury. *Seminars in Neonatology* **5**, 3-16.

Inder TE, Huppi PS, Warfield S, Kikinis R, Zientara GP, Barnes PD, Jolesz F, Volpe JJ (1999) Periventricular white matter injury in the premature infant is followed by reduced cerebral cortical gray matter volume at term. *Annals of Neurology* **46**, 755-760.

Ischiropoulos H, Zhu L, Chen J, Tsai M, Martin JC, Smith C, and Beckman JS (1992) Peroxynitrite-mediated tyrosine nitration catalyzed by superoxide dismutase. *Archives of Biochemistry and Biophysics* **298**, 431-437.

Inselman LS, Fisher SE, Spencer H, Atkinson M (1985) Effect of intrauterine ethanol exposure on fetal lung growth. *Pediatric Research* **19**, 12–14.

Ishihara N, Matsuo H, Murakoshi H, Laoag-Fernandez J, Samoto T, Maruo T (2000) Changes in proliferative potential, apoptosis and Bcl-2 protein expression in cytotrophoblasts and syncytiotrophoblast in human placenta over the course of pregnancy. *Endocrine Journal* **47**, 317-327.

Jackson I T, Hussain K (1990) Craniofacial and oral manifestations of fetal alcohol syndrome. *Plastic and Reconstructive Surgery* **85**, 505-512.

Jacobson MD (1996) Reactive oxygen species and programmed cell death. *Trends in Biochemical Sciences* **21**, 83- 86.

Jaenisch R, Bird A (2003) Epigenetic regulation of gene expression: how the genome integrates intrinsic and environmental signals. *Nature Genetics* **33**, 245–254.

Jansson T, Powell T (2007) Role of the placenta in fetal programming: underlying mechanisms and potencial interventional approaches. *Clinical Science* **113**, 1–13.

Jones KL, Smith DW (1973) Recognition of the fetal alcohol syndrome in early infancy. *Lancet* **2**, 999-1001.

Jones KL, Smith DW, Ulleland CN, Streissguth AP (1973) Pattern of malformations in offspring of chronic alcoholic mothers. *Lancet* **1**, 267-271.

Kasina S, Rizwani W, Radhika KV, Singh SS (2005) Nitration of profilin effects its interaction with poly (L-proline) and actin. *Journal of Biochemistry* **138**, 687-695.

Kasina S, Wasia R, Fasim A, Radhika KV, Singh SS (2006) Phorbol ester mediated activation of inducible nitric oxide synthase results in platelet profilin nitration. *Nitric Oxide* **14**, 65-71.

Kattainen H, Tuukkanen J, Simanainen U, Tuomisto JT, Kovero O, Lukinmaa PL, Alaluusua S, Tuomisto J, Viluksela M (2001) In utero/lactation 2,3,7,8-tetrachlordibenzo-p-dioxin exposure impairs molar tooth development an rats. *Toxicology and Applied Pharmacology* **174**, 216-224.

Kaufman MH (1992) *The Atlas of Mouse Development*. pp 1-512. London: Academic Press.

Villamor E, Kessels CGA, van Suylen RJ, Jo G.R. De Mey Jo GR, Blanco. (2005) Cardiopulmonary effects of chronic administration of the NO Synthase Inhibitor L-NAME in the Chick Embryo. *Biology of the Neonate* **88**,156–163.

Kay HH, Grindle KM, Magness RR (2000) Ethanol exposure induces oxidative stress and impairs nitric oxide availability in the human placental villi: A possible mechanism of toxicity. *American Journal of Obstetrics and Gynecology* **182**, 682-688.

Kingdom JC, Kaufmann P (1999) Oxygen and placental vascular development. *Advances in Experimental Medicine and Biology* **474**, 259-275.

Komuro H, Rakic P (1994) Identification of membrane proteins that comprise the plasmalemmal junction between migrating neurons and radial glial cells. *Journal of the Neurological Sciences* **18**, 1478-1490.

Komuro H, Rakic P (1998) Orchestration of neuronal migration by activity of ion channels, neurotransmitter receptors, and intracellular Ca2+ fluctuations. *Journal of Neurobiology* **37**, 110-130.

Kossenjans W, Eis A, Sahay R, Brockman D, Myatt L (2000) Role of peroxinitrite in altered fetal-placental vascular reactivity in diabetis or preeclampsia. *American Journal of Physiology. Heart and Circulatory Physiology* **278**, H311-H319.

Kotch LE, Chen SY, Sulik KK (1995) Ethanol-induced teratogenesis : free radical damage as a possible mechanism. *Teratology* **52**, 128-136.

Kumada T, Jiang Y, Cameron DB, Komuro H (2007) How does alcohol impair neuronal migration? *Journal of Neroscience Research* **85**, 465-470.

Kumar A, Singh CK, DiPette DD, Singh US (2010) Ethanol impairs activation of retinoic acid receptors in cerebellar granule cells in a rodent model of fetal alcohol spectrum disorders. *Alcoholism, Clinical and Experimental Research* **34**, 928-937.

Lazic T, Wyatt TA, Matic M, Meyerholz DK, Grubor B, Gallup JM, Kersting KW, Imerman PM, Almeida-De-Macedo M, Ackermann MR (2007) Maternal alcohol ingestion reduces surfactant protein. A expression by preterm fetal lung epithelia.
Alcohol **41**, 347-355.

Lazic T, Sow FB, Van Geelen A, Meyerholz DK, Gallup JM, Ackermann MR (2011) Exposure to ethanol during the last trimester of pregnancy alters the maturation and immunity of the fetal lung. *Alcohol* **45**, 673–80.

Lee YH, Spuhler-Phillips K, Randall PK, Leslie SW (1994) Effects of prenatal ethanol exposure on N-methyl-Daspartate-mediated calcium entry into dissociated neurons. *Journal of Pharmacology and Experimental Therapeutics* **271**, 1291-1298.

Leers MP, Kolgen W, Bjorklund T, Tribbick G, Persson B, Bjorklund P, Ramaekers F C, Bjorklund P, Nap M, Jornvall H, Schutte B (1999) Immunocytochemical detection and mapping of a Cytokeratin 18 neo-epitope exposed during early apoptosis. *Journal of Pathology* **187**, 567-572.

Lefkowitch JH, Rushton AR, Feng-Chen KC (1983) Hepatic fibrosis in fetal alcohol syndrome. Pathologic similarities to adult alcoholic liver disease. *Gastroenterology* **85**, 951-957.

Levy R, Smith SD, Yusuf K, Huettner PC, Kraus FT, Sadovsky Y, Nelson DM (2002) Trophoblast apoptosis from pregnancies complicated by fetal growth restriction is associated with enhanced p53 expression. *American Journal of Obstetrics and Gynecology* **186**, 1056-1061.

Liochev SI, Fridovich I (1997) How does superoxide dismutase protect against tumor necrosis factor: a hypothesis informed by effect of superoxide on "free" iron. *Free Radical Biology and Medicine* **23**, 668- 671.

Liu X, Zou H, Slaughter C, Wang X (1997) DFF, a heterodimeric protein that functions downstream of caspase-3 to trigger DNA fragmentation during apoptosis. *Cell* **89**, 175-184.

Lockhart EM, Warner DS, Pearlstein RD, Penning DH, Mehrabani S, Boustany RM (2002) Allopregnanolone attenuates N-methyl- D - aspartate-induced excitotoxicity and apoptosis in the human NT2 cell line in culture. *Neuroscience Letters* **328**, 33-36.

Loser H, Pgeferkorn J R, Themann H (1992) Alcohol in pregnancy and fetal heart damage. *Klinische Pädiatrie* **204**, 235-239.

Luciana M (2003) Cognitive development in children born preterm: implications for theories of brain plasticity following early injury. *Development and Psychopathology* **15**, 1017-1047

MacMillan-Crow LA, Thompson JA (1999) Tyrosine modifications and inactivation of active site manganese superoxide dismutase mutant (Y34F) by peroxynitrite. *Archives of Biochemistry and Biophysics* **366**, 82-88.

Magistretti PJ (2006) Neuron-glia metabolic coupling and plasticity. *Journal of Experimental Biology* **209**, 2304-2311 Review

Maier SE, Chen WJ, Miller JA, West JR (1997) Fetal alcohol exposure and temporal vulnerability regional differences in alcohol-induced microencephaly as a function of the timing of binge-like alcohol exposure during rat brain development. *Alcoholism, Clinical and Experimental Research* **21**, 1418-1428.

Mankes RF, LeFevre R, Fieseher J, Santiago A, Benitz KF, Lyon R (1985) Effects of ethanol on reproduction and arterial hypertension in spontaneously hypertensive and normotensive rats: a preliminary communication. *Alcoholism, Clinical and Experimental Research* **9**, 284-290.

Malatesta P, Hartfuss E, Gotz M (2000) Isolation of radial glial cells by fluorescent-activated cell sorting reveals a neuronal lineage. *Development* **127**, 5253-5263.

Martin SJ, Reutelingsperger CP, McGahon AJ, Rader JA, Schie RC van, LaFace DM, Green DR (1995) Early redistribution of plasma membrane phosphatidylserine is a general feature of apoptosis regardless of the initiating stimulus: inhibition by overexpression of Bcl-2 and Abl. *Journal of Experimental Biology* **182**, 1545-1556.

Matsubara S, Sato I (2001) Enzyme histochemically detectable NAD(P)H oxidase in human placental trophoblast: normal, preeclamptic, and fetal growth restriction-complicated pregnancy. *Histochemistry and Cell Biology* **116**, 1-7.

Mattson SN, Riley EP (1998) A review of the neurobehavioral deficits in children with fetal alcohol syndrome or prenatal exposure to alcohol. *Alcoholism, Clinical and Experimental Research* **22**, 279-294.

Mauceri HJ, Lee WH, Conway S (1994) Effect of ethanol on insulin-like growth factor-II release from fetal organs. *Alcoholism, Clinical and Experimental Research* **18**, 35–41.

Michaelis EK (1990) Fetal alcohol exposure: cellular toxicity and molecular events involved in toxicity. *Alcoholism, Clinical and Experimental Research* **14**, 819-826.

Miller DK (1997) The role of the caspase family of cysteine proteases in apoptosis. *Seminars in Immunology* **9**, 35-40.

Miller MW, Potempa G (1990) Numbers of neurons and glia in mature rat somatosensory cortex: effects of prenatal exposure to ethanol. *Journal of Comparative Neurology* **293**, 92-102.

Miller MW (1996) Effect of early exposure to ethanol on the protein and DNA contents of specific brain regions in the rat. *Brain Research* **734**, 286-294.

Millet C, Lemaire P, Orsetti B, Guglielmi P, Francois V (2001) The human chordin gene encodes several differentially expressed spliced variants with distinct BMP opposing activities. *Mechanisms of Development* **106**, 85–96.

Mitchell JA, Goldman H. (1996) Effects of alcohol on blastocyst implantation site blood flow in the rat. *Alcohol & Alcoholism,*. **31**, 81-87.

Montoliu C, Sancho-Tello M, Azorin I, Burgal M, Valles S, Renau-Piqueras J, Guerri C (1995) Ethanol increases cytochrome P4502E1 and induces oxidative stress in astrocytes. *Journal of Neurochemistry* **65**, 2561-2570.

Morimoto M, Zern M A, Hagbjork AL, Ingelman-Sundberg M, French SW (1994) Fish oil, alcohol, and liver pathology: role of cytochrome P450 2E1. *Proceedings of the Society for Experimental Biology and Medicine* **207**, 197-205.

Morris-Kay G (1993) Retinoic acid and craniofacial development: molecules and morphogenesis. *Bioessay* **15**, 9-15.

Myatt L, Brewer AS, Langdon G, and Brockman DE (1992) Attenuation of the vasoconstrictor effect of thromboxane and endothelin by nitric oxide in the human fetal placental circulation. *American Journal of Obstetrics and Gynecology* **16**, 224-230.

Myatt L, Rosenfield LD, Eis AL, Brockman DE, Greer E, Lyall F (1996) Nitrotirosine residues in placenta. Evidence of peroxinitrite formation and action. *Hypertension* **28**, 488-493.

Myatt, L., Eis, A. L., Brockman, D. E., Kossenjans, W., Greer, I., & Lyall, F (1997) Inducible (type II) nitric oxide synthase in human placental villous tissue of normotensive, pre-eclamptic and intrauterine growthrestricted pregnancies. *Placenta* **18**, 261-268

Myatt L (2002) Role of placenta in preeclampsia. *Endocrine* **19**, 103-111.

Myatt L, Cui X (2004) Oxidative stress in the placenta. *Histochemistry and Cell Biology* **122**, 369-382.

Myatt L (2006) Placental adaptive responses and fetal programming. *Journal of Physiology* **572**, 25–30.

Myatt L (2010) Review: reactive oxygen and nitrogen species and functional adaptation of the placenta. *Placenta* **31**, S66-S69.

Myllynen P, Pasanen M, Pelkonen O (2005) Human placenta. A human organ for developmental toxicology research and biomonitoring. *Placenta* **26**, 361-371.

Nakatsuji N, Johnsson K E (1984) Effects of ethanol on the primitive streak stage mouse embryo. *Teratology* **29**, 269-275.

Nasser MI, Lee HI, Kim MO (2010) Neuroprotective effect of vitamin C against the ethanol and nicotine modulation of $GABA_B$ receptor and PKA-α expression in prenatal rat brain. *Synapse* **64**, 467-477.

Nelissen EC, van Montfoort AP, Dumoulin JC, Evers JL (2011) Epigenetics and the placenta. *Human Reproduction Update* **17**, 397–417.

Neumann P, Gertzberg N, Vaughan E, Weisbrot J, Woodburn R, Lambert W, Johnson A (2006) Peroxynitrite mediates TNF-α-induced endothelial barrier dysfunction and nitration of actin. *American Journal of Physiology. Lung Cellular and Molecular Physiology* **290**, L674-L684.

Newmeyer DD, Ferguson-Miller S (2003) Mitochondria: releasing power for life and unleashing the machineries of death. *Cell* **112**, 481-490.

Nissen MD (2007) Congenital and neonatal pneumonia. *Paediatric Respiratory Reviews* **8**, 195–203

Noctor SC, Flint AC, Weissman TA, Dammerman RS, Kriegstein AR (2001) Neurons derived from radial glial cells establish radial units in neocortex. *Nature* **409**, 714-720.

Ochs, M (2006) A brief update on lung stereology. *Journal of Microscopy* **222**, 188– 200.

Oh SI, Kim CI, Chun HJ, Park SC (1998) Chronic ethanol consumption affects glutathione status in rat liver. *Journal of Nutrition* **128**, 758-763.

Olney J W, Wosniak D F, Farber N B, Jevtovic-Todorovic V, Bittigau P, Ikonomidou C (2002) The enigma of fetal alcohol neurotoxicity. *Annals of Medicine* **34**, 109-119.

Ornoy A (2007) Embryonic oxidative stress as a mechanism of teratogenesis with special emphasis on diabetic embryopathy. *Reproductive Toxicology* **24**, 31-41.

Oyedele O, Kramer B (2013) Nuanced but significant: How ethanol perturbs avian cranial neural crest cell actin cytoskeleton, migration and proliferation. *Alcohol* **47**, 417-426.

Pacher P, Beckman JS, Liaudet L (2007) Nitric oxide and peroxynitrite in health and disease. *Physiological Reviews* **87**, 315-424.

Palacios-Callender M, Quintero M, Hollis VS, Springett RJ, Moncada S (2004) Endogenous NO regulates superoxide production at low oxygen concentrations by modifying the redox state of cytochrome *c* oxidase. *Proceedings of the Society for Experimental Biology and Medicine* **101**, 7630–7635.

Paoletti AM, Romagnino S, Contu R, Orru MM, Marotto MF, Zedda P, Lello S, Biggio G, Concas A, Melis GB (2006) Observational study on the stability of the psychological status during normal pregnancy and increased blood levels of neuroactive steroids with GABA-A receptor agonist activity. *Psychoneuroendocrinology* **31**, 485–492.

Pijnenborg R, Bland JM, Robertson WB, Dixon G, Brosens I (1981a) The pattern of interstitial trophoblastic invasion of the myometrium in early human pregnancy. *Placenta* 2, 303-316.

Pijnenborg R, Robertson WB, Brosens I, Dixon G (1981b) Review article: trophoblast invasion and the establishment of haemochorial placentation in man and laboratory animals. *Placenta* 2, 71-91

Plessinger MA, Woods JR, Miller RK (2000) Pretreatment of human amnion-chorion vitamin C and E prevents hypoclorous acid-induced damage. *American Journal of Obstetrics and Gynecology* **183**, 979-985.

Qanungo, S., Mukherjea, M (2000) Ontogenic profile of some antioxidants and lipid peroxidation in human placental and fetal tissues. *Molecular and Cellular Biochemistry* **215**, 11-19.

Radi R, Beckman JS, Bush KM, Freeman BA (1991). Peroxynitrite-induced membrane lipid peroxidation: the cytotoxic potential of superoxide and nitric oxide. *Archives of Biochemistry and Biophysics* **288**, 481-487.

Radi R, Beckman JS, Bush KM, Freeman BA (1994) Inhibition of mitochondrial electron transport by peroxinitrite. *Archives of Biochemistry and Biophysics* **308**, 89-95.

Radi R, Cassina A, Hodara R (2002) Nitric oxide and peroxynitrite interactions with mitochondria. *Biological Chemistry* **383**, 401-409.

Radi R, Beckman JS, Bush KM, Freeman BA (1991) Peroxynitrite-induced membrane lipid peroxidation: the cytotoxic potential of superoxide and nitric oxide. *Archives of Biochemistry and Biophysics* **288**, 481-487.

Rakic P (1972) Mode of cell migration to the superficial layers of fetal monkey neocortex. *Journal of Comparative Neurology* **145**, 61-83.

Rakic P (1995) Radial versus tangential migration of neuronal clones in the developing cerebral cortex. *Proceedings of the National Academy of Sciences of the United States of America* **92**, 11323-11327.

Randall CL, Taylor WJ (1979) Prenatal ethanol exposure in mice: Teratogenic effects. *Teratology* 19:305–312.

Reik W, Constancia M, Fowden A, Anderson N, Dean W, Ferguson-Smith A, Tycko B, Sibley C (2003) Regulation of supply and demand for maternal nutrients in mammals by imprinted genes. *Journal of Physiology* **547**, 35–44.

Reinke LA, Lai EK, DuBose CM, McCay BP (1987) Reactive free radical generation in vivo in heart and liver of ethanol-fed rats: correlation with radical formation in vitro. *Proceedings of the National Academy of Sciences of the United States of America* **84**, 9223-9227.

Renaul-Piqueras J, Guasch R, Azorin I, Segul JM, Guerri C (1997) Prenatal alcohol exposure affects galactosyltransferase activity and glycoconjugates in the Golgi apparatus of fetal rat hepatocytes. *Hepatology* **25**, 343-350.

Rodrigo R, Parra M, Bosco C, Fernández V, Barja P, Guajardo J, Messina R (2005) Pathophysiological basis for the prophylaxis of preeclampsia through early supplementation with antioxidant vitamins. *Pharmacology & Therapeutics* **107**, 177-97.

Rosenberg MJ, Wolff CR, El-Emawy A, Staples MC, Perrone-Bizzozero NI, Savage D D (2010) Effects of moderate drinking during pregnancy on placental gene expression. *Alcohol* **44**, 673-690.

Rosset HL (1980) A clinical perspective of the fetal alcohol syndrome. *Alcoholism-Clinical and Experimental Research* **4**, 119-122.

Rout UK, Dhossche JM (2010) Liquid-diet with alcohol alters maternal, fetal and placental weights and the expression of molecules involved in integrin signaling in the fetal cerebral cortex. *International Journal of Environmental Research and Public Health* **7**, 4023-4036.

Rubert G, Miñana R, Pascual M, Guerri C (2006) Ethanol exposure during embryogenesis decreases the radial glial progenitor pool and affects the generation of neurons and astrocytes. *Journal of Neuroscience Research* **84**, 483-496.

Sandor GS, Smith DF, Mac Leod PM. (1981) Cardiac malformations in the fetal alcohol syndrome. *Journal of Pediatrics* **98**, 771-773.

Salihu HM, Kornosky JL, Lynch O, Alio AP, August EM, Marty P (2011) Impact of prenatal alcohol consumption on placenta-associated syndromes. *Alcohol* **45**, 73-79.

Sant'Anna LB, Tosello DO (2006) Fetal alcohol syndrome and developing craniofacial and dental structures-a review. *Orthodonties and Craniofacial Research* **9**, 172-185.

Schumacher M, Guennoun R, Stein DG, De Nicola AF (2007) Progesterone: therapeutic opportunities for neuroprotection and myelin repair. *Pharmacology & Therapeutics* **116**, 77-106.

Seppa K, Laippala P, Sillanaukee P (1996) High diastolic blood pressure: Common among women who are heavy drinkers. *Alcoholism-Clinical and Experimental Research* **20**, 47-51.

Senftleben U, Cao Y, Xiao G, Greten FR, Krahn G, Bonizzi G, Chen Y, Hu Y, Fong A, Sun SC, Karin M (2001) Activation by IKKalpha of a second, evolutionary conserved, NF-kappa B signalling pathway. *Science* **293**, 1495-1499.

Sies H (1991) Role of reactive oxygen species in biological processes. *Wiener Klinische Wochenschrift* **69**, 965-968.

Shaukat A, Champagne D, Alia A, Richardson M (2011) Large-Scale Analysis of Acute Ethanol Exposure in Zebrafish Development: A Critical Time Window and Resilience. *Public Library of Science* **6**, e20037:1-16.

Shi H, Noguchi N, Xu Y, Niki E (1999) Formation of phospholipid hydroperoxides and its inhibition by alpha-tocopherol in rat brain synaptosomes induced by peroxynitrite. *Biochemical and Biophysical Research Communications* **257**, 651-656.

Smith SC, Baker PN, Symonds EM (1997) Placental apoptosis in normal human pregnancy. *American Journal of Obstetrics and Gynecology* **177**, 57-65.

Smith SM (1997) Alcohol-induced cell death in the embryo. *Alcohol Health and Research World* **21**, 287-297.

Soares MJ (2004) The prolactin and growth hormone families: pregnancy-specific hormones/cytokines at the maternal fetal interface. *Reproductive Biology and Endocrinology* **2**, 51-66.

Sozo F, Dick AM, Bensley JG, Kenna K, Brien JF, Harding R, De Matteo R (2013) Alcohol exposure during late ovine gestation alters fetal liver iron homeostasis without apparent dysmorphology. *American Journal of Physiology, Regulatory, Integrative and Comparative Physiology* **304(12)**, R1121-R1129.

Sozo F, O'Day L, Maritz G, Kenna K, Stacy V, Brew N, Walker D, Bocking A, Brien J, Harding R (2009) Repeated ethanol exposure during late gestation alters the maturation and innate immune status of the ovine fetal lung. *American Journal of Physiology Lung Cellular and Molecular Physiology* **296**, L510–L518.

Sulik KK (1984) Critical period for alcohol teratogenesis in mice, with special reference to the gastrulation stage of embryogenesis. *Ciba Foundation Symposium* **105**, 124-141.

Sulik KK, Johnston MC, Webb MA (1981) Fetal alcohol syndrome: Embryogenesis in a mouse model. *Science* (Wash. DC) **214**, 936–938.

Szabo C, Zingarelli B, O'Connor M, Salzman AL (1996) DNA strand breakage, activation of poly (ADPribose) synthetase, cellular energy depletion are involved in the cytotoxicity of macrophages and smooth muscle cells exposed to peroxynitrite. *Proceedings of the National Academy of Sciences of the United States of America* **93**, 1753-1758.

Szabó C (2003) Multiple pathways of peroxynitrite cytotoxicity. *Toxicology Letters* **140**, 105-112.

Taléns-Visconti R, Sanchez Vera I, Kostic J, Perez-Arago MA, Erceg S, Stojkovic M, Guerri C (2011) Neural differentiation from human embryonic stem cells as a tool to study early brain development and the neuroteratogenic effects of ethanol. *Stem Cells Development* **20**, 327-339.

Taylor SM, Heron AE, Cannell GR, Florin TH (1994) Pressor effect of ethanol in the isolated perfused human placental lobule. *European Journal of Pharmacology* **270**, 371-374.

Tedeschi G, Cappelletti G, Negri A, Pagliato L, Maggioni MG, Maci R, Ronchi S (2005) Characterization of nitroproteome in neuron-like PC12 cells differentiated with nerve growth factor: identification of two nitration sites in alpha-tubulin. *Proteomics* **5**, 2422-2432.

Temple S (2001) The development of neural stem cells. *Nature* **414**, 112-117.

Terrapon M, Schneider P, Friedli B, Cox JN (1977) Aortic arch interruption type A with aortopulmonary fenestration in an offspring of chronic alcoholic mother ("fetal alcohol syndrome"). *Helvetica Pediatric Acta* **32**, 141-148.

Thomas JD, Abou EJ, Dominguez HD (2009) Prenatal choline supplementation mitigates the adverse effects of prenatal alcohol exposure on development in rats. *Neurotoxicology and Teratology* **31**, 303–311

Tran TD, Kelly SJ (2003) Critical periods for ethanol-induced cell loss in the hippocampal formation. *Neurotoxicology and Teratology* **25**, 519-528.

Tran TD, Jackson HD, Hom KH, Goodlett CR (2005) Vitamin E does not protect against neonatal ethanol-induced cerebellar damage or deficits in eyeblink classical conditioning in rats. *Alcoholism-Clinical and Experimental Research* **29**, 117-129.

Villamor E, Kessels CG, van Suylen RJ, De Mey JG, Blanco CE (2005) Cardiopulmonary effects of chronic administration of the NO synthase inhibitor L-NAME in the chick embryo. *Biology of the Neonate* **88(3)**, 156-63.

Virag L, Szabo E, Gergely P, Szabo C (2003) Peroxynitrite-induced cytotoxicity: mechanism and opportunities for intervention. *Toxicology Letters* **140**, 113-124.

Wang X, Gomutputra P, Wolgemuth DJ, Baxi L (2007) Effects of acute alcohol intoxication in the second trimester of pregnancy on development of the murine fetal lung. *American Journal of Obstetrics and Gynecology* **197**, 269 e1.–269. e4.

Watson AL, Palmer ME, Jauniaux E, Burton GJ (1997) Variations in expression of copper/zinc superoxide dismutase in villous trophoblast of the human placenta with gestational age. *Placenta* **18**, 295-299.

Webster RP, Roberts VH, Myatt L (2008) Protein nitration in placenta: functional significance. *Placenta* **29**, 985-994.

Wells PG, Ma Callum GP, Chen CS, Henderson JT, Lee CLL, Perstin J, Preston TJ, Wiley MJ, and Wong AW (2009) Oxidative stress in developmental origins of disease: teratogenesis, neurodevelopmental deficits, and cancer. *Toxicological Sciences* **108**, 4-18.

Wentzel P, Eriksson UJ (2008) Genetic influence on dysmorphogenesis in embryos from different rat strains exposed to ethanol in vivo and in vitro. *Alcoholism-Clinical and Experimental Research* **32**, 874-887.

Wentzel P, Eriksson UJ (2009) Altered gen expression in neural crest cells exposed to ethanol in vitro. *Brain Research* **1305**, S50-S60.

Wentzel P, Rydberg U, Eriksson UJ (2006) Antioxidative treatment diminishes ethanol-induced congenital malformations in the rat. *Alcoholism-Clinical and Experimental Research* **30**, 1732-1760.

West JR, Kelly SJ, Pierce DR.(1987) Severity of alcohol-induced deficits in rats during the third trimester equivalent is determined by the pattern of exposure. *Alcohol and Alcoholism Supplement* **1**, 461-465

Yawno T, Yan EB, Walker DW, Hirst JJ (2009) (2007) Inhibition of neurosteroid synthesis increases asphyxia-induced brain injury in the late gestation fetal sheep. *Neuroscience* **146**, 1726-1733.

Yui J, Hemmings D, Garcia-Lloret M, Guilbert LJ (1996) Expression of the human p55 and p75 tumor necrosis factor receptors in primary villous trophoblasts and their role in cytotoxic signal transduction. *Biology of Reproduction* **55**, 400-409.

Zhou F, Zhao Q, Liu Y, Goodlett C, Liang T, McClintick J, Edenberg H, Li L (2011) Alteration of gene expression by alcohol exposure at early neurulation. *Bio Medical Central Genomics* **12**, 124-141.

Zou MH., Leist M, Ullrich V (1999) Selective nitration of prostacyclin synthase and defective vasorelaxation in atherosclerosic bovine coronary arteries. *American Journal of Pathology* **54**, 1359-1365.

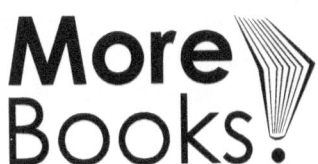

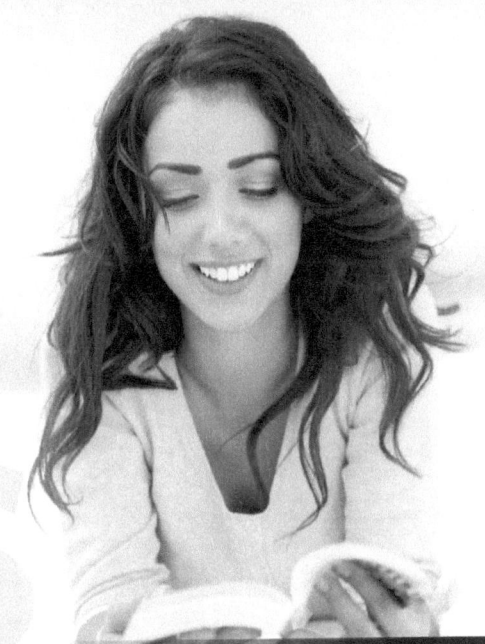

i want morebooks!

Buy your books fast and straightforward online - at one of world's fastest growing online book stores! Environmentally sound due to Print-on-Demand technologies.

Buy your books online at

www.get-morebooks.com

Kaufen Sie Ihre Bücher schnell und unkompliziert online – auf einer der am schnellsten wachsenden Buchhandelsplattformen weltweit! Dank Print-On-Demand umwelt- und ressourcenschonend produziert.

Bücher schneller online kaufen

www.morebooks.de

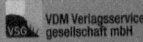 VDM Verlagsservicegesellschaft mbH
Heinrich-Böcking-Str. 6-8 Telefon: +49 681 3720 174 info@vdm-vsg.de
D - 66121 Saarbrücken Telefax: +49 681 3720 1749 www.vdm-vsg.de

www.ingramcontent.com/pod-product-compliance
Lightning Source LLC
Chambersburg PA
CBHW031545210526
45464CB00003B/1152